Sexual
Reflexology

Sexual Reflexology

Activating the Taoist Points of Love

Mantak Chia and William U. Wei

Destiny Books
Rochester, Vermont

Destiny Books
One Park Street
Rochester, Vermont 05767

Destiny Books is a division of Inner Traditions International

ISBN 0-89281-088-2

Printed and bound in the United States of America

Text design by Cynthia Ryan Coad
This book was typeset in Janson, with Diotima as a display typeface

Putting Sexual Reflexology into Practice

The practices described in this book have been used successfully for thousands of years by Taoists trained by personal instruction. It is preferable that readers do not undertake these practices without receiving personal transmission and training from a certified instructor of the Universal Tao, since some of these practices, if done improperly, may cause injury or result in health problems. Universal Tao Instructors can be located at the Universal Tao website: www.universal-tao.com or www.taoinstructors.org.

This book is intended to supplement individual training in the Universal Tao and to serve as a reference guide for these practices. Anyone who undertakes these practices solely on the basis of this book alone does so entirely at his or her own risk.

The meditations, practices, and techniques described herein are not intended to be used as an alternative or substitute for professional medical treatment and care. If any readers are suffering from illnesses based on mental or emotional disorders, an appropriate professional health-care practitioner or therapist should be consulted. Such problems should be corrected before training begins.

Neither the Universal Tao nor its staff and instructors can be responsible for the consequences of any practice or misuse of the information contained in this book. If the reader undertakes any exercise without strictly following the instructions, notes, and warnings, the responsibility must lie solely with the reader.

This book does not attempt to give any medical diagnosis, treatment, prescription, or remedial recommendation in relation to any human disease, ailment, suffering, or physical condition whatsoever.

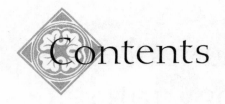

Contents

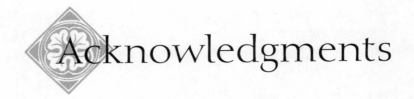

Acknowledgments

The Universal Tao Publications staff involved in the preparation and production of *Sexual Reflexology: Activating the Taoist Points of Love* extends gratitude to the many generations of Taoist masters who have passed on their special lineage, in the form of an oral transmission, over thousands of years. We thank Taoist master I Yun (Yi Eng) for his openness in transmitting the formulas of Taoist Inner Alchemy.

Thanks to Juan Li for the use of his beautiful and visionary paintings illustrating Taoist esoteric practices.

We offer our eternal gratitude to our parents and teachers for their many gifts to us. Remembering them brings joy and satisfaction to our continued efforts in presenting the Universal Tao system.

As always, their contribution has been crucial in presenting the concepts and techniques of the Universal Tao.

We wish to thank the thousands of unknown men and women of the Chinese healing arts who developed many of the methods and ideas presented in this book.

We express special thanks to Lee Holden for his writing and editorial contributions. We appreciate his research and great labor. We express deep appreciation to Mamo for his illustrations. We thank Karen Holden and Lisa Yamamoto for their assistance in preparing, editing, and proofreading the manuscript. We wish to thank Colin Campbell, DeAnna Satre, Vickie Trihy, and Robert Marsh for their editorial contributions in the revised edition of this book.

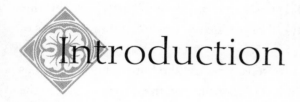 # Introduction

The Taoists have written and taught on the subject of sexual energy for the last five thousand years. This book is part of a series written to pass on some of this precious information, and to shed light on how to create positive fulfilling relationships in your life. By combining the classic Taoist sexual texts with modern reflexology theory, *Sexual Reflexology* can enable any individual or couple to better understand their sexual energy and to cultivate that energy for health and well-being.

FOOT REFLEXOLOGY

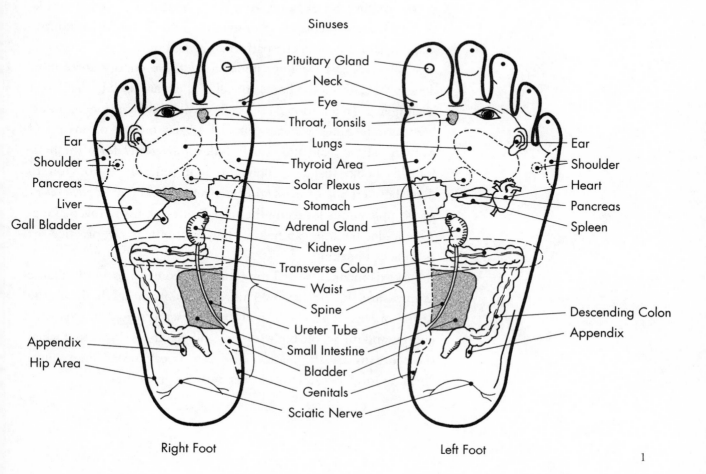

Sinuses

Pituitary Gland
Neck
Eye
Throat, Tonsils
Lungs
Thyroid Area
Solar Plexus
Stomach
Adrenal Gland
Kidney
Transverse Colon
Waist
Spine
Ureter Tube
Small Intestine
Bladder
Genitals
Sciatic Nerve

Ear
Shoulder
Pancreas
Liver
Gall Bladder

Appendix
Hip Area

Ear
Shoulder
Heart
Pancreas
Spleen

Descending Colon
Appendix

Right Foot

Left Foot

When most people hear the term *reflexology*, they think of foot massage. In the West, it is common to see charts, like the one below, that map out the areas of the body correlating to regions of the feet.

Charts like this make sense because the human body begins as a single cell that contains a blueprint for the entire body. As the body grows, energy meridians run through it and key parts of the body are mapped over and over again, based on the original blueprint. Rather like a hologram, a three-dimensional picture in which every part contains the whole, each part of the body has a mapping for the entire body. These energetic mappings are regularly used in Oriental medicine and are beginning to be more accepted in the West.

Reflexology is based on the premise that all our organs have reflex points on other parts of the body. The corresponding points are found by dividing the body into different zones. Organs in a particular zone can be stimulated by working on reflexes in the corresponding reflex-point zone. The meridians used in traditional Oriental medicine, acupuncture, and shiatsu also indicate mappings of the energetic pathways in the body.

The Taoists have long understood these energy correspondences throughout the body, and all of them are used in the Taoist healing arts. In addition to the reflexes already mentioned, Taoist literature includes reflexes for the sexual organs of men and women. These male and female reflexology zones form the basis for this book. Just as a book on foot reflexology goes on to describe methods of massaging the reflexes, so *Sexual Reflexology* gives applications for using the sexual reflex points in lovemaking. This understanding can help couples and individuals practice sex as an act of healing.

In this manner, sexual intercourse becomes a form of ecstatic acupressure. The most powerful reflex points on the body are the sexual organs. The whole body provides the sexual organs with energy, and the whole body (organs and glands) is stimulated when these organs are stimulated. The Taoists call sexual intercourse "healing love" because of its deep healing properties.

THE UNIVERSAL TAO

Taoist practice aims at aligning ourselves with the structure of the universe. The first step in connecting with the universe is to establish a harmonious relationship with ourselves. It is through the inner journey of meditation that the Taoists come to know themselves. This is the goal of the Universal Tao, an extensive system of self-development and spiritual cultivation. Using this system, we harmonize all our seemingly separate parts—emotions, thoughts, physical body, and spiritual aspirations—with a variety of Taoist techniques. Exploring the system as a whole provides a full spectrum of life enhancing skills, in which sexual health is an essential part. Sexual reflexology is an important component of the system.

Universal Tao Instructors are available in the Americas to teach you Master Chia's Universal Tao System of Chi Kung (qi gong) and Nei Kung for physical, emotional, and spiritual cultivation. Each instructor has been personally trained by Mantak Chia and the Universal Tao family of teachers. Ongoing classes, workshops, private instruction, private healing sessions, video and audio products, and retreats are available to people of all ages and conditions of health. Universal Tao centers are available in most major cities, and continuing education credits may be available. To contact a local instructor in your area visit our website: www. universal-tao.com, www.taoinstructors.org, or call (888) 444-7426.

The Healing Love Practice

The Healing Love practice of the Universal Tao refers to the cultivation of sexual energy. Sexual reflexology is an intricate aspect of the Healing Love practice. Healing Love utilizes sexual energy for the health of the body, mind, and spirit. There are practices for single cultivation (by oneself) and dual cultivation (with a partner). This book will demonstrate and discuss a variety of Healing Love practices that will bring health and vitality into your life and into your relationships. It will describe diagnostic techniques to reveal compatibility between male and female partners and also present specific exercises (sexercises) that strengthen our sexual imbalances and weaknesses. These exercise postures bring health, vitality, and an abundance of energy to those who practice them.

THE IMPORTANCE OF MEDITATION IN SEXUAL REFLEXOLOGY

The following preliminary meditation from the Universal Tao is called the Microcosmic Orbit. It develops inner strength and harmony, which are indispensable requirements for a fulfilling relationship with another person. It is recommended that you also regularly practice the Inner Smile and Six Healing Sounds meditations, to transform negative emotions and stress into beneficial energy. These two techniques are fully explained in my book *Transform Stress into Vitality*.

Microcosmic Orbit

The first step in working with internal energy is the Microcosmic Orbit meditation. This meditation trains one to sense, direct, and cultivate more energy. This technique is the core of all the other Universal Tao practices. The Microcosmic Orbit is the main energetic circuit, nourishing all the channels and meridians in the body—the "super-highway" for the Chi (energy). Circulating energy within this channel removes blockages and activates more Chi to revitalize the body. Through this practice, one learns to recognize what Chi feels like while moving energy through two important energy channels in the body. The first channel, called the Functional, or Conception, meridian, begins at the base of the trunk in the perineum, midway between a man's testicles or a woman's vaginal opening and the anus. It goes up the front of the body past the genitals, stomach, heart, and throat and ends at the tip of the tongue. The second channel, the Governor meridian, begins in the same place but goes up the back of the body—into the tailbone, up through the spine, into the brain and back down through the roof of the mouth. The tongue is like a switch that connects these two currents—when it is touched to the roof of the mouth just behind the front teeth, the energy can flow in a circle up the spine and back down the front of the body. Thus the two channels form a single circuit that the energy loops around. This vital current, called the Microcosmic Orbit, circulates past the major organs and nervous system, giving cells the juice they

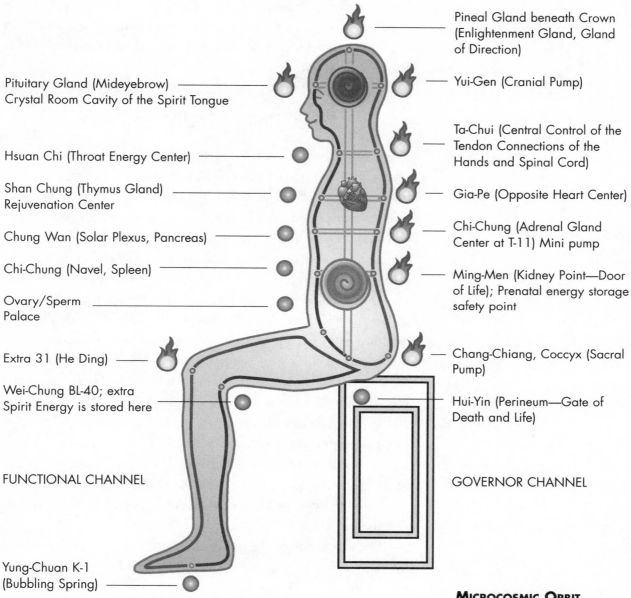

Pineal Gland beneath Crown (Enlightenment Gland, Gland of Direction)

Pituitary Gland (Mideyebrow) Crystal Room Cavity of the Spirit Tongue

Yui-Gen (Cranial Pump)

Ta-Chui (Central Control of the Tendon Connections of the Hands and Spinal Cord)

Hsuan Chi (Throat Energy Center)

Shan Chung (Thymus Gland) Rejuvenation Center

Gia-Pe (Opposite Heart Center)

Chung Wan (Solar Plexus, Pancreas)

Chi-Chung (Adrenal Gland Center at T-11) Mini pump

Chi-Chung (Navel, Spleen)

Ming-Men (Kidney Point—Door of Life); Prenatal energy storage safety point

Ovary/Sperm Palace

Extra 31 (He Ding)

Chang-Chiang, Coccyx (Sacral Pump)

Wei-Chung BL-40; extra Spirit Energy is stored here

Hui-Yin (Perineum—Gate of Death and Life)

FUNCTIONAL CHANNEL

GOVERNOR CHANNEL

Yung-Chuan K-1 (Bubbling Spring)

MICROCOSMIC ORBIT

need to grow, heal, and function. The Microcosmic Orbit meditation dramatically increases the quantity of our internal energy.

To open the microcosmic energy channel, sit in meditation, preferably after doing the Inner Smile meditation. Allow your energy to complete the loop by letting your mind flow along with it. Start in the eyes, and mentally circulate with the energy as it goes down the front through your tongue, throat, chest, and navel, and then up the tailbone and spine to the head. This is different from visualizing an image inside your head of what that part of the body looks or feels like. Do not use your mind like a television camera. Relax and let your mind flow with the Chi in the physical body along its natural circuit.

DIRECTING SEXUAL ENERGY

When improperly directed, the sex impulse can be so strong and compelling that people will risk all they have, including their reputation and freedom, in order to express this drive. When this force is transmuted and directed in a positive way, however, it can be used as a powerful creative force in any endeavor that is being pursued, whether in the arts, in a career or profession, in a loving relationship, or in just developing a strong, magnetic personality.

The human is the only animal who has the ability to direct sexual energy with his or her imagination whenever desired. The only question is: How is it going to be directed? Some choose to use this energy in abusive and negative ways; some merely waste it and disperse it indiscriminately by overindulging. There are many ways in which we can express this energy, both positively and negatively. With the proper guidance, the sexual energy can be a rich treasure of joy, happiness, and passion. It can be a tool to create and maintain optimum health and vitality, transforming a mediocre life into an exceptional one, changing a stress-filled, unhappy life into one filled with success and fulfillment. It is simply that powerful.

The vibrations of the mind are easily increased and activated by many different types of stimuli. The mind responds easily to love, deep friendships, music, as well as fear, jealously, drugs, alcohol, and the like. But the most intense stimulus is the desire to express sexual energy. When combined with love, sexual energy is the most powerful stimulus of all and remains a virtue only to the degree that it is used discriminately, with wisdom, compassion, and understanding. With this understanding comes a responsibility to use the extra energy gained in loving and positive ways. This is the only way to create a rich and fulfilled life.

Nothing is more important than relationships. To establish harmonious relationships in all aspects of life is the goal of the

Taoist practice. The universe, nature, and the world we live in operate through relationships, connections, and social exchange. To establish harmonious, balanced relationships is the process of the Tao; it is the balance of all apparent opposites, male and female, light and darkness, rest and activity, electricity and magnetism.

The Taoist yin-and-yang symbol is a representation of this balance and harmony. The male and female energies of nature are always moving toward balance. The Taoists observed that the way of nature is interactive and full of creative, life-giving, sexual energy. Rain penetrates the earth, giving birth to trees and flowers; rivers caress rocks; the ocean plunges into the sand; and the sunshine is absorbed into the womb of the earth, giving birth to all life. Sexual energy is the creative force that permeates the universe. Life springs forth from balancing male and female energies, through the combination of yin and yang. These same principles apply to human relationships. Sexual reflexology is about discovering balance and harmony within ourselves and in our relationships.

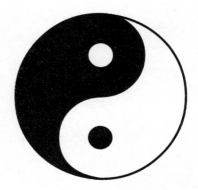

YIN AND YANG— FEMALE AND MALE

SPECIAL NOTE FOR WOMEN READERS

Please, while reading this book, be aware of two things:

1. The practices described originate in a society vastly different from most modern societies. China was an overwhelmingly male-dominated society in which men possessed the political, civil, and monetary power and women had little or no opportunity for independent action or existence. While evidence of this imbalance may remain in some of the language and postures of the ancient Taoist literature represented here, it is intended that the contents of this book be used to provide equal and mutual benefits for women and men.

2. This book has been written by two authors who are themselves male, and therefore it may seem to reflect sexuality from the standpoint of a man. Nonetheless, it is our genuine intention to help demystify the female nature for our readers, and to assist couples to achieve a deeper understanding of one another's physical and spiritual needs.

Male and Female Energy

Her eyebrows are like a bouquet of flowers; her waist is like a roll of silk. With tender passion she stretches out furtively and she gazes coyly at her own body. They first pat and knead their flexed bodies and caress each other from head to toe.

—Po Hsing-Chien (from a ninth-century erotic essay)

It is important to understand the difference between male sexual energy (yang) and female sexual energy (yin). The Taoists understood that men and women are meant to balance, as two opposite halves of a universal whole. This means that we need to respect our differences and understand that it is natural to feel different and to be different. Without this awareness men and women are often at odds with one another. Many of our struggles in relationships come about because we expect each other to be the same. I hear many people complain that their partner does not see things the way they do, or does not do things the way they do. It is important not to fight and struggle with our differences but to make them work in our favor, creating balance and harmony. If we forget this truth, we are easily upset and frustrated with the opposite sex. Yet when we respect this difference, love blossoms like a well-nurtured garden. Sexual reflexology is designed to harmonize these male and female challenges on an energetic level.

Sexually, men are like fire, quick to get hot and quick to explode. Women, on the other hand, are like water, heating up slowly and staying hot longer. This is the reason male Taoists use a variety of techniques to satisfy a woman sexually. Women need foreplay, to be caressed tenderly and embraced with passion. This way the water, the feminine sexual energy, will boil and energy will be exchanged. Thus the Taoist saying "Never sail your boat in a rocky river," meaning that the woman needs to be aroused and lubricated before sexual intercourse.

In cultivating sexual energy, men learn to control ejaculation and achieve a full-body orgasm rather than merely a genital orgasm. By learning to transform sperm into Chi, men can become better lovers, more vibrant and youthful, and are able to activate the compassionate energy in the heart. For women, cultivating sexual energy is a way to transform blood into Chi. Transforming sexual energy is directly related to the menstrual cycle. From the Taoist exercises, this transformation leads to an abundance of energy, balanced emotions, and internal power. For a detailed description of these techniques, refer to my books *The Multi-Orgasmic Man* and *Taoist Secrets of Love: Cultivating Female Sexual Energy*.

Emotionally, women are like fire and men are like water. It is

BELOW LEFT: WOMEN CHANGE BLOOD INTO CHI

BELOW RIGHT: MEN CHANGE SEMEN INTO CHI

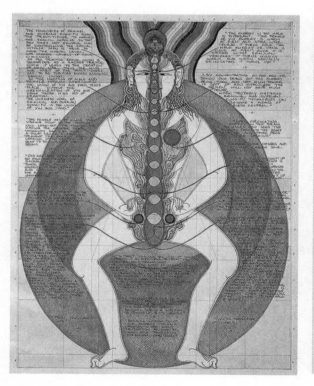

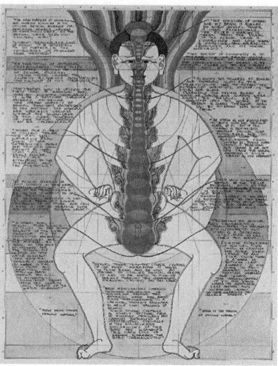

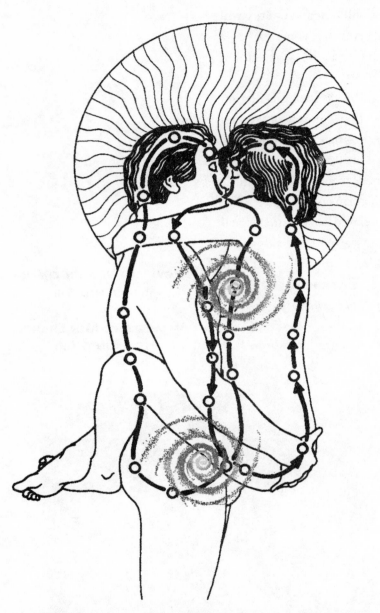

FUSION OF THE TWO MICROCOSMIC ORBITS AND THE SEXUAL AND HEART CENTERS

very easy for women to express their emotions, to get excited, to cry, and to feel. For men it is more challenging to be in touch with the heart center. This is how men and women balance emotionally and sexually. Women open and heat the emotional center, or the heart center, in men, and men help open or bring fire into the sexual center for women. The goal of the Taoist practice is to create this harmonious and flowing exchange of energy.

This is revealed physically by the fact that men project from the sexual center (the penis) and women project from the heart center (the breasts). Projection is the yang or the fire quality of energy. This demonstrates that women are yang emotionally and men are yang sexually. These physical features reveal the energetic and emotional nature of men and women.

YIN AND YANG

The "tractor" (yang) and the "lake" (yin) are the energy fields of the man and of the woman. We are speaking of opposites: when the man is hot, the woman is cold; when the woman is hot, the man is cold. So you have a real communication problem. When you're very hot, the person with whom you are trying to communicate is cold. Men and women have different types of energy molecularly. It's very hard to communicate unless you have a clear understanding of your own energy field and how it interacts with the people around you, especially the energy field of the opposite gender. Getting this understanding opens up communication, which is the key to any relationship.

"The tractor and the lake" exemplifies what I mean by this difference. When you drive a tractor into a lake, you get stuck. And what happens when the tractor tries to fight the lake? It sinks deeper. Who is stronger, the tractor or the lake? Obviously, the lake is stronger. It not only has its own energy but also absorbs all of the energy the tractor exerts. Now, the tractor is active energy and the lake is passive energy. The lake is the yin energy, or the feminine energy, and the tractor is the yang, or the male, energy. So the woman is far superior to the man in every aspect: physically, emotionally, psychologically, and spiritually. Physically, from the waist down, a woman is far superior to a man. She can outwork a man. She lives longer and has more strength in her lower body.

In endurance of pain and physical hardships she far exceeds the man. Her body is structurally far superior to the man's body. Emotionally she works with more of her feelings and has a stronger capacity with her emotional center. Psychologically she tunes in to her inner self with telepathy and clairvoyance. A woman is more apt to make this connection than a man because of her physical structure. Because her genitals are internal, a woman is disposed to access her internal world, whereas a man's genitals are external, making him more externally oriented. A woman is more spiritually attuned than a man because of the inner connection with herself and her understanding of and connection with the earth energy, nature.

The key message in "the tractor and the lake" is the ability of the lake to yield to the tractor, and the way of the Tao is to yield because the Tao is feminine. You find this in every aspect. Every time you want to overcome something, you yield to its energy and you use its energy for your own benefit and welfare.

The following is a story giving an example of how the genders move towards either an external (to resist) or internal (to yield)

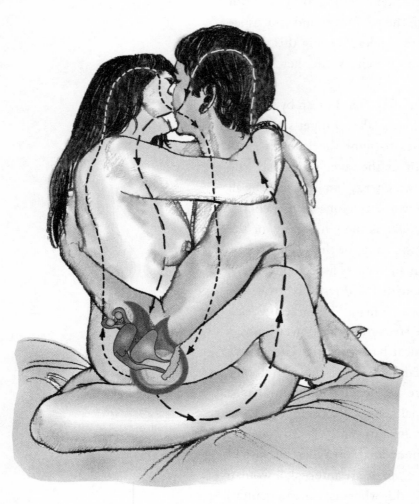

MALE FIRE ENERGY TO HEAT THE FEMALE EGGS

perspective. When children are born, both genders have to urinate. The male child has all of his equipment down there and he can see everything. He can see his equipment and urinates out. His outlook in life is external because his focus is external. But when the little girl urinates, she's looking to find where it is coming from. She's looking inside herself because she doesn't see anything down there. She's curious about what's inside her. Through spaced repetition, many times urinating and many times puzzling over this issue, she begins to look and feel what's inside her.

The male proceeds through life and looks at everything externally. It's all right there. He takes control of his genital area. He becomes the master of it. He understands it and comes in contact with it. The woman, on the other hand, doesn't come into contact with the genitals because they aren't there. They're inside her body. Because they're inside, she is drawn to look inside her body. As she matures as an adolescent, she begins to form breasts and she begins to get in touch with her chest area, thus getting in touch with her heart center, which is the center of the emotions and the feeling center. She starts to work directly with these emotions and feelings. This difference affects the genders' outlook on life: As a woman internalizes, she personalizes or she takes things personally; as a man externalizes, he generalizes or talks in generalities. You can see this has a major impact on how they live and how they communicate with each other, which leads to confusion and differences.

The man seldom touches himself in the chest area. He never gets in touch with his heart center. He never gets in touch with his feelings or his emotions. The woman becomes the master of the emotions and the male becomes the master of the sexual energy or the kidney energy. But each can help the other. An example of this is what I call "boiling eggs."

You put two eggs in a pan of hot water and you put them on the burner to boil. The male can get an erection, or start the fire, just like that! But it takes a while for the woman to warm up, just as it takes a while for those eggs to warm up. She needs some foreplay. She needs to be caressed. She needs her eggs warmed up. The eggs in her body, her kidney energy, have to be activated at a slow pace and brought to a boil slowly. The male's sexual energy normally can turn on and off quickly. But once the man understands how the woman's energy functions and learns many of the Universal Tao techniques (such as the shallow thrusting technique), he'll maintain his fire at a lower temperature so she can build to her climax, boiling the eggs. As her eggs start to boil, she achieves her orgasm, but she also needs to come down slowly. That's why women like a lot of caressing, holding, and being with their partner many hours after genital interaction, just as you need to cool the eggs down.

The funniest thing about this whole scenario is that the same thing is needed for the heart energy but in reverse. The woman can turn her emotions on and off just as quickly as a man can turn his kidney (sexual) energy on and off. She has so much experience working with her feelings in her heart center. She can help a man to get in touch with his feelings and heart center. She has to caress with emotional foreplay, developing and nurturing the man so that he can get in touch with his feelings. Many times, when a man gets in touch with his feelings, he needs to come down slowly (just as she needs to with her kidney energy) to cool the eggs off, or to

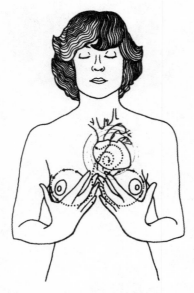

ABOVE: WARMING THE CAULDRON IN THE HEART CENTER

BELOW: WU CHI (ONENESS) INTO YIN/YANG (DUALITY)

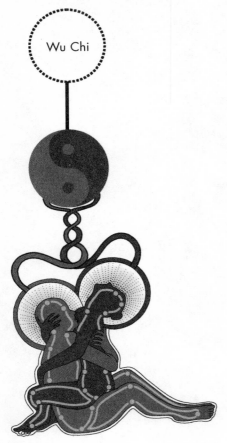

Wu Chi

cool the heart off, so that he can get in touch with it. So both genders, once they understand their energy fields and how they interact, can help develop a nice harmony with one another by helping each other. The key to the interaction between the genders is communication, and this means connecting with the heart energy.

Taoists really don't look at sex or the use of sexual energy as a moral issue. It's more of a health issue. Once you begin to understand your energy, what it is about and what it is actually for, you can have a much healthier understanding of how to work with it and how it interacts with everyone around you, especially with the opposite gender. The best way to explain this is dual cultivation. Taoist practices lend themselves to a monogamous relationship similar to playing a doubles tennis match. You have a partner on your team. You learn your partner's form, how he or she interacts. It takes many years to develop good rapport and a good understanding of each other's moves. The same thing occurs in the Taoist interaction of sexual energies. Once you have a partner in dual cultivation, it takes many years to perfect a nice harmony. And you don't want to switch your partner, just like you don't want to switch your partner in a tennis doubles match, because you have to learn again all the various moves and techniques of a new partner. The same concept applies in the Tao with dual cultivation.

Just as you practice tennis, your serve and forehand, in singles to help your partner in the doubles, you start to practice the single cultivation aspects in order to be ready for dual cultivation. You need to perfect the techniques of the Universal Tao system with Testicle Breathing and Ovarian Breathing, as well as Genital Compression, and the Big or Upward Draw technique. (Please reference *The Multi-Orgasmic Man* and *Healing Love Through the Tao: Cultivating Female Sexual Energy* for thorough descriptions on the latter two practices.) Testicle Breathing and Ovarian Breathing transform raw sexual energy to a higher energy to nourish the spine, the nervous system, the brain, and the organs. These practices increase the energy in the brain and the nervous system tremendously.

To practice Testicle Breathing, sit relaxed on the edge of a chair with genitals unsupported. Massage the testicles for a few minutes. Contract very slightly first the left testicle and draw this energy up to the tailbone and then up through the sacrum and spine to the brain. You can follow the Microcosmic Orbit instructions from here. Always remember to place your tongue to the roof of your mouth to allow the energy to return to your Lower Tan Tien. Repeat with the right testicle. At first it may seem like nothing is happening, but keep practicing with intention and you will start to feel the energy from the testicle rise up.

To practice Ovarian Breathing, sit relaxed on the edge of a chair with genitals unsupported (women should have the genitals covered). Find your ovaries and rub them until warm. Contract and release the vagina; then contract the vagina and contract very slightly the left ovary, drawing this energy down through the uterus and back wall of the vagina to the perineum, and then up to the tailbone, through the sacrum and spine to the left brain. You can follow the Microcosmic Orbit instructions from here. Always remember to place your tongue to the roof of your mouth to allow the energy to return to your Lower Tan Tien. This is especially important for women as the unaroused sexual energy is the hot energy and should not be left in the brain. Repeat with the right ovary. As with the men, at first you may not notice anything happening. Just keep practicing with intention and you will start to feel the energy from the ovaries rise up.

As you work with these techniques and thus balance the energy internally on a chemical level, you're going to begin to attract a more balanced partner. You should really focus on working primarily with the heart energy, to balance yourself internally with love, compassion, and patience, becoming at peace and in harmony within yourself. The key is communication, because the tongue is connected to the heart. You have to explain how you feel, who you are, and where you want to go. With this open and honest communication, you and your partner will discover whether you are compatible with each other, sharing the intent to assist each other in your spiritual journeys.

The Taoists say, "Sex is like an itch. It feels good when you scratch it, but it feels better when you do not have the itch." When you develop this balance, you're going to start to attract a person who will be a potential spiritual helpmate and life partner.

The key to the Taoists' sexual practices is "chicken soup."

When you make chicken soup, you put a chicken and water in a pot and boil it. After two hours you take the chicken out and you have the broth. Now, what would you rather eat, the chicken or the broth? The broth, because it has all the essence of the chicken in it. The same with the sexual practices: The chicken is your genitals and the broth is your sexual essence. When you cook (Testicle Breathing and Ovarian Breathing and the Upward Draw practices) the chicken (genitals) and draw the broth (essence) up your spine into the brain, you have a brain orgasm instead of a genital orgasm. Now, the brain is connected to all parts of the body, giving a total body orgasm. So, which would you rather have, a chicken (genital) orgasm or a broth (essence) brain orgasm? Think about it: the chicken and the broth.

This procedure of extracting the sexual essence from the genitals and moving it up into the body is further developed in the Universal Tao formulas of the Healing Love dual cultivation practice, looking into each other's eyes, exchanging healing cosmic energy like magnets. Dual Cultivation should start with both partners having their Microcosmic Orbits open. The couple then exchange sexual energy in their Microcosmic Orbits during lovemaking. This balancing and nourishing exchange of yin and yang energies is the heart of the Healing Love practice and part of what eventually leads the dedicated student beyond sexual pleasure to longevity.

There is one very important fact that you have to understand about the genders when they interact. When a man is sexually aroused he is jet hot (a fire burning), but when a woman is sexually aroused she is icy cold (a numb burning). When a man is sexually unaroused he is cool (relaxed), but when a woman is sexually unaroused she is warm (cozy). They are opposites. Men understand this hot aroused feeling quite easily. Women also feel a hot sensation, but it is a different type of hot, like the sensation of an ice cube burning your skin, which numbs the skin. This sensation leaves the woman feeling helpless. That is why a woman is very vulnerable in this aroused state, because she loses control of herself; in the same way, the man loses control of his feelings when he opens his heart center.

This basic difference between the genders manifests itself on all levels of consciousness. That is why they find it very hard to read and understand each other. They do not think alike; the man thinks with logic and the woman thinks with feeling. Men think methodically: One and one is two, not eleven. They are very structured and predictable; ultimately they become prisoners of their own mind. Women actually think correctly, using their sense of heart direction with their feelings, as one would think in the Tao. But they run into trouble when they mix up their feelings with their out of balance emotions, and they miss the target. There is a big difference between a feeling and an emotion: A feeling is a direction from the heart center (God), and an emotion is a sensation from an imbalanced organ.

As you can see, it is surprising, with all these differences, that men and women ever get together at all. It is easy to understand why they have so many problems when they do get together. But if they are compatible, they have a great opportunity to develop divine love, as spiritual helpmates to one another on the journey into nothingness.

Sexual Energy:
A Taoist Perspective

Sexual energy is nourishment for the totality of ourselves—the body, the mind, and the spirit. It is the water of life, replenishing the gardens of the human temple. The exercises for sexual energy developed in the Taoist teachings are much more sophisticated and focused than in the West, where sexual cultivation is not very advanced and there are no real techniques for developing or understanding the sexual energy They go right to the source of our sexuality and cultivate it in a way that brings sexual energy and strength to those who use them properly.

The philosophy of Chi has been part of the Chinese culture for thousands of years. The word *Chi* has many translations, such as energy, air, breath, life force, or vital essence. It is the life-giving force that creates movement and sustains the universe. Chi is what allows planets, suns, and stars to revolve around each other. It is the motion of the atom in all physical bodies. It is the force that allows a seed to grow into a powerful tree or a fetus into a full-grown human being. Chi is the animating factor in all living things, nourishing the cycles of life.

The concepts of energy are not only food for thought but concrete ways in which we can create health, happiness, and excitement in our daily lives. Working with energy is a pivotal factor in our overall state of happiness. Energy, like water, is the life-giving sustenance of the earth. Where water flows, life flourishes. That same principle is at work in our bodies. If we want a healthy body, energy must circulate to all parts. Without proper energy flow, the body creates tension, sickness, and disease. It is like a stagnant pool or a dried-up garden. Without continuous circulation, things have a tendency to become malignant.

Thus sexual energy, according to the Taoists, is much more than the act of sex, because it permeates all areas of our lives. It influences the health and aging of the body by affecting hormonal production. An abundance of sexual energy repairs hormonal disturbances, reduces cholesterol, and decreases blood pressure levels. When sex glands are stimulated, it enhances the hormones secreted by the other major endocrine glands: adrenal, thymus, thyroid, pituitary, and pineal. Much evidence points to the link between harmonious sexual activity and the retardation of aging. Sexual reflexology stimulates the growth hormones, whose abilities to retard aging are just now being discovered by Western medicine. In the Taoist perspective, hormones should be stimulated naturally, through exercises and massage, not taken externally through medication. The presence of these hormones in the blood does appear to slow the aging process. With Taoist cultivation of sexual energy techniques, one produces unusually potent hormones by focusing energy directly on the endocrine glands. Sexual energy is not only beneficial to the body but fuels the emotions as well, which can either blaze out of control or create warm, comfortable, glowing energy in the body. Sexual imbalances can cloud the mind with distorted thoughts and skewed desires, but a balanced sexuality can be the source of creativity and a way of fulfilling our dreams. It is also the energy that can create spiritual fulfillment, as it is a force that unifies and creates wholeness out of opposites.

From this perspective, we can begin to see that it is of utmost importance that we deal with and utilize sexual energy. It is very important to remember that sexual energy must be used in the proper way and not be suppressed or eliminated. Suppressing sexual energy is like trying to hold hundreds of Ping-Pong balls underwater. If you press them down, they pop up somewhere else. Instead, sexual reflexology seeks to express this energy in a way that will enhance your body, mind, and spirit. Otherwise this energy will seek outlets through which it will be underutilized and wasted or could even be potentially detrimental to one's overall health. Whether you have a partner or not, the ideas and exercises in this book are vitally important to sexual health. The Taoists developed these techniques so that we can live in harmony with ourselves and others.

We have compiled a variety of techniques that will most definitely increase the sexual energy of those who engage in these practices. The practices have a profound effect on the rest of our lives because our sexuality is so much a part of being human. There is so much power behind our sexuality that without the proper knowledge of how to manage and direct that energy, it will inevitably go astray. Yet with the correct knowledge and balanced action, our sexual energy has the potential to bring happiness and joy into all aspects of our lives. It is essential that we as human beings tap into our true potential, gaining the insight to create a passionate and powerful life and become all that we are meant to be.

SEXUALITY, ENERGY, AND RELATIONSHIPS

The relationship between men and women has baffled and confused philosophers, scientists, and thinkers throughout the ages. Sexuality is a dance that spans the history of all societies. It is a ritual that has preoccupied the activities of humankind throughout the aeons and still has present cultures in a quandary. For something that has existed for so long and has been a part of everyone's life throughout history, one would think that humanity would have some expertise on the subject of sexuality. Yet to this very day, our sexual relationships continue to daze and confuse the spirit of people in profound ways. On the one hand they create passion and love, ignite romance and pleasure, and spark the flames of desire that make life worth living. But on the other hand, sexuality is also a source of destruction and negativity that are the causes of a myriad of problems in society.

Sex is a creative force that moves through the body, feeding the emotions and thoughts and creating the impulse of desire. It is pleasure in its raw and unrefined state. If that energy is not understood and used in the right way, it is the cause of dissatisfaction, destruction, and overall unhappiness in our lives. As basic as the

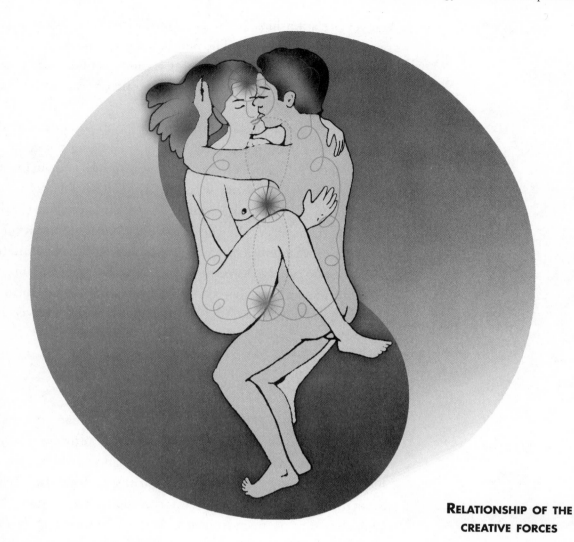

**RELATIONSHIP OF THE
CREATIVE FORCES**

duality of man and woman, day and night, sexual energy can be the source of both pain and pleasure.

Sexuality is like the force of fire. When used intelligently, it enhances our lives immensely. With fire we can warm our houses, cook our food, and bring light into dark rooms. But if we use fire in the wrong way, for example, putting it on the roof instead of in the fireplace, it will inevitably burn the whole house down. The fire itself is not evil or even bad, it is merely a force that needs to be directed in a positive way. The same applies with sexuality; if we use it correctly, it brings us unbelievable pleasure, but if we let this energy run wild without guidance or understanding, it has the potential to destroy our physical and emotional lives.

Not only is there an overall dissatisfaction with sex in our everyday relationships, but we are faced with the malicious acts of rape, abuse, and violence. The number of problems in society that revolve around the topic of sexuality is monumental. The echoing question of how to use this energy in positive ways can be heard throughout the world.

In the tradition of Taoism, sex was seen in an altogether different context than in the West. Rather than being the great sin, sexual energy was considered a path toward health and vitality and a way to connect intimately with the divine. That divinity is seen as a state of wholeness and completeness that is implicit in all of us. In the traditions of the East, man and woman represent opposite halves of that universal whole. Each is an earthly manifestation of the cosmic creative forces—yin and yang, feminine and masculine, Heaven and Earth—whose intermingling brings forth all phenomena. When man and woman unite in sex, Heaven and Earth are joined.

HISTORY OF SEXUAL REFLEXOLOGY

For thousands of years, Taoists have explored human potential in relation to sexuality. The knowledge acquired provides a way to enhance relationships, sexual energy, pregnancy, birthing, vitality, and the health of body, mind, and spirit. The legendary Yellow Emperor (second century B.C.E.) recorded conversations with Taoist advisors on many subjects. The works *Classic of the Plain Girl* (Arcane Maid*)* and *Counsels of a Simple Girl* are recorded conversations on sexual matters. These recordings give a great deal of information on the use of sexual energy to achieve vibrant health and longevity. These ancient classics are a treasure chest of information on all issues dealing with sexuality. *Sexual Reflexology* is a reflection of some of this wisdom.

The following information regarding the determination of sexual inclination, capacity, and functioning of human beings has a specific purpose in Taoist sexology. From ancient times and until recently in China, many marriages were arranged by parents. The information they used to determine compatibility and suitability of partners was researched with great care and love, and the result was often a very happy and fulfilled marital relationship. Although women have had the right to divorce in China for at least a thousand years, this was a rare occurrence, possibly because everything was so carefully considered in advance. Information used in selecting a compatible marriage partner was quite complete, including factors such as personality, physical compatibility, and family circumstances as well as individual intelligence, education, and social status as determined by Chinese astrology and reflexology. Reviewing the marital union with such care and great detail resulted in a high likelihood for compatibility in the partnership. With this approach, the strength, love, and unity of the family group was greatly enhanced. Considering the exceptionally high divorce rates in Western society today, the valuable information that is provided by such an approach could prove helpful. The unhappiness and emotional difficulties experienced by both parents and children involved in marriage dissolution in our modern society are immeasurable.

While almost any kind of assistance to improve this situation would be useful, the Taoist time-proven system of reviewing a range of important compatibility factors cannot be overlooked as useful to the appropriate union of a man and woman. If a man and woman were able to choose a suitable sexual partner, resulting in their greater mutual happiness, this method will have served its purpose. It is with an attitude of reverence for the sanctity of marriage and the union between men and women that this idea of researching compatibility factors is offered.

UNION OF SEXUAL COMPATIBILITY

Reflexology

In their search into the art of lovemaking, the ancient Chinese Taoists went beyond foods and herbs, even beyond erotic techniques . . . by consciously maneuvering the human body's Chi, or life-energy. They did this to enhance sexual arousal, control orgasm and intensify ecstasy for both men and women.

VALENTIN CHU, YIN-YANG BUTTERFLY

Reflexology has traditionally been practiced by massaging and pressing points on the hands and feet. These techniques have been proven to be a powerful method of healing. Yet reflexology is much more extensive than merely pressure points on the hands and feet. *Reflexology* refers to reflection, or mirror image. The Taoist sages learned to use external physical features to learn about internal energy, health of the organs, and personality. Reflexology teaches that vital energy, or life force, circulates among the organs and every living tissue in the body. Sexual reflexology uses ancient Taoist wisdom to tap in to a rich source of vitality by working with sexual energy and the way it manifests in the body. It is based on the principle that sexual health is an indispensable aspect of a fulfilling life. Discovering the spring of sexual potential within is a way to access the abundance of energy inside us.

In traditional Chinese Taoist medicine, various diagnostic methods recognize a physical connection between a person's external appearance (physiognomy)—particularly the visible characteristics of the hands and face—and the size, shape, and condition of his or her internal organs. It is also believed that various parts of our physical anatomy are directly proportional in size and shape to one another. Thus, a relationship is established between the size and shape of external features, the condition of internal features, and a proportionate correspondence with all the features on the body. This principle is considered a law of anatomy, which Taoist physicians know and practice as a science and art, now popularly called reflexology.

Consider how the following external features are used to diagnose the health of the internal organs. The eyes reflect the liver: Are they bright or cloudy, do they have occlusions or spots, and so on? A healthy liver will be reflected by a clear, deeply colored iris with no spots, scars, blurry areas, or the like. The lips reflect the spleen, the nose reflects the lungs, the ears reflect the kidneys, and the tip of the nose and aspects of the tongue reflect the heart. Color, texture, clarity, and so on are the conditions of these external features that directly reflect the health of the internal organ with which they are associated by the meridians, or energy lines, from the organs to the extremities of the body.

While single external features are an indication of sexual potential (a larger thumb indicates a larger penis), it is the combination of many external features that reveals the true sexual potential. It is an art to be skilled at these diagnostic techniques and it takes many years of training to develop. Using these diagnostic techniques can be very beneficial in revealing our strengths and weaknesses. Once we know ourselves, we can begin to balance those areas that are weak and need extra energy. This way we become a much more complete and unified human being. The Taoists always recommend discovering and improving our weaker areas to promote overall balance.

COMPATIBILITY OF THE PENIS AND VAGINAL CANAL

Man and woman should ebb and flow in intercourse like the waves and currents of the sea. In this manner, they may continue all night long, constantly nourishing and preserving their precious vital essence, curing all ailments and promoting long life.

—SUN NU CHING (THE CLASSIC OF THE PLAIN GIRL)

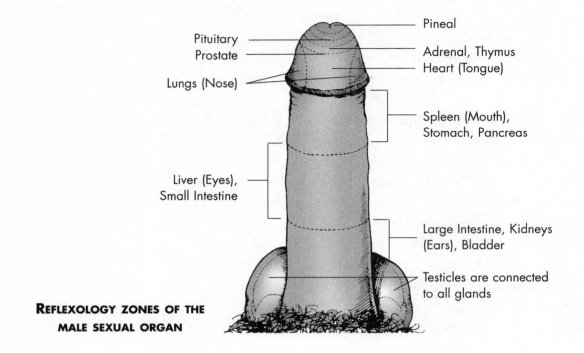

Pineal

Pituitary

Prostate

Adrenal, Thymus
Heart (Tongue)

Lungs (Nose)

Spleen (Mouth),
Stomach, Pancreas

Liver (Eyes),
Small Intestine

Large Intestine, Kidneys
(Ears), Bladder

Testicles are connected
to all glands

**REFLEXOLOGY ZONES OF THE
MALE SEXUAL ORGAN**

**REFLEXOLOGY ZONES OF
THE FEMALE SEXUAL ORGAN**

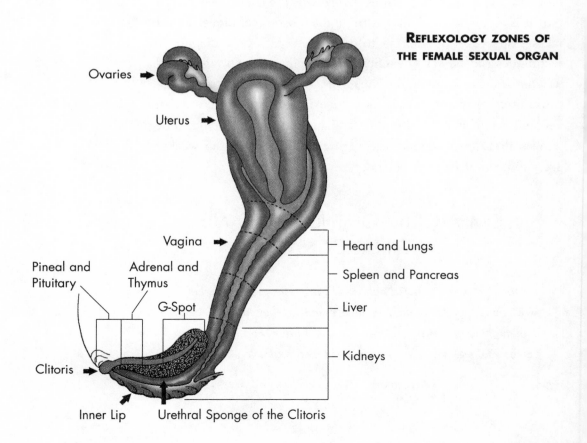

Ovaries ➤

Uterus ➤

Vagina ➤

Heart and Lungs

Spleen and Pancreas

Pineal and
Pituitary

Adrenal and
Thymus

G-Spot

Liver

Kidneys

Clitoris ➤

Inner Lip   Urethral Sponge of the Clitoris

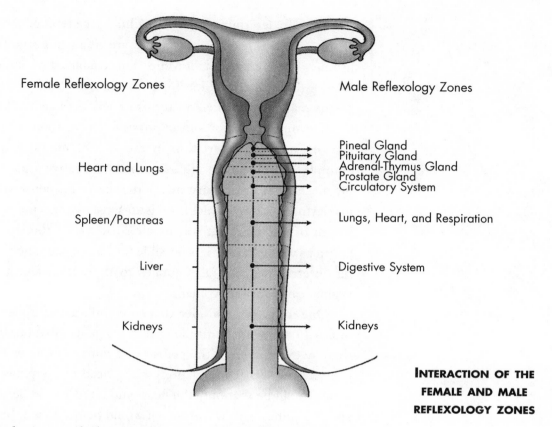

Female Reflexology Zones

Male Reflexology Zones

Heart and Lungs

Pineal Gland
Pituitary Gland
Adrenal-Thymus Gland
Prostate Gland
Circulatory System

Spleen/Pancreas

Lungs, Heart, and Respiration

Liver

Digestive System

Kidneys

Kidneys

**INTERACTION OF THE
FEMALE AND MALE
REFLEXOLOGY ZONES**

Taoist sexologists teach that sexual intercourse is a form of ecstatic acupressure. The ends of the body are a rich source of acupressure and reflex points, which is why reflexology is usually applied to the feet, hands, ears, or face. Yet the most intense and powerful reflex points on the body are the sexual organs themselves. Sexual energy is derived from the best energy of the body. The whole body is involved with providing the sexual center with energy. Therefore the sexual center is the condensation of all the body's energy. This is the reason that the health of the sexual center is critical to our mental, emotional, and physical health.

When the sexual organs of the male and female unite, a wonderful stimulation of energy is experienced through the whole body. Sexual intercourse is an ecstatic acupressure treatment. The Taoists call sexual intercourse "healing love" because of its deep healing properties. Ancient Taoist physicians even prescribed certain sexual positions to couples in order to stimulate the sexual reflexology points in a particular way.

Sexual reflexology also helps determine compatibility between partners. To determine this compatibility, the level of sexual desire and the physical features of the body are vitally important in establishing a harmonious relationship. This enables the couple's sexual relationship to be fulfilling for both partners. Such compatibility means matching partners in terms of sexual capacity, desire, and the size and proportion of the physical organs themselves. There may be substantial variation in the size of men's genitalia, for example. This is neither a positive nor a negative aspect but simply means that a man must match the size of his penis with that of his partner's vaginal canal if he is to satisfy her completely. If the length of the man's penis is much greater than the length of his partner's vaginal canal, it is possible for him to cause her harm during intercourse. This also applies to the length and size of the vaginal canal for the woman.

One must also consider that to completely stimulate a man's internal organs, the entire length of his penis must be stimulated, thereby exciting all of the penis reflex zones. If one were to concentrate the sexual stimulation on the head of the penis only, the result would be that only the heart and lungs would be stimulated and the kidneys, liver, and spleen would be neglected. In time this would result in an imbalance—the heart and lungs being overactivated and the liver, spleen, and kidneys underactivated.

A similar situation exists in the vaginal canal. For a woman to be completely stimulated internally, that is, to ensure equal stimulation of her vital organs, the man's penis must reach to the end of the vaginal canal. It is recognized in Taoist sexology that the flexibility or elasticity of a woman's vaginal canal is relatively small in relationship to its length; however, it has much greater flexibility in width, demonstrated by the fact that the vaginal canal can expand to accommodate a baby traveling through it from the womb during childbirth. Thus we can see that compatibility of length is more important than compatibility of width. The resultant pleasure of such compatibility leads to sexual fulfillment.

RING MUSCLES

The ancient Taoists discovered the subtle and intricate power of the ring muscles within the body. The ring muscles are the round

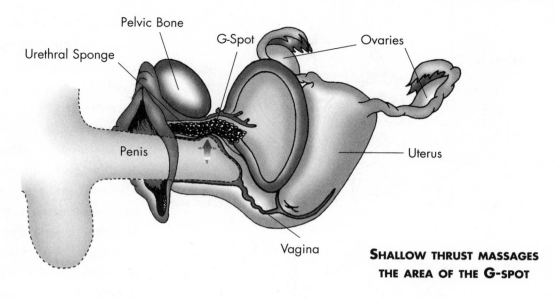

Pelvic Bone

Urethral Sponge

G-Spot

Ovaries

Penis

Uterus

Vagina

SHALLOW THRUST MASSAGES THE AREA OF THE G-SPOT

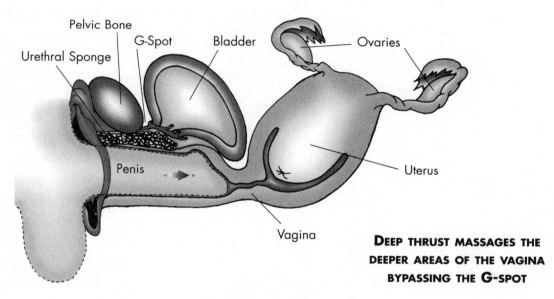

Pelvic Bone

Urethral Sponge

G-Spot

Bladder

Ovaries

Penis

Uterus

Vagina

DEEP THRUST MASSAGES THE DEEPER AREAS OF THE VAGINA BYPASSING THE G-SPOT

sphincter muscles of the mouth, eyes, nostrils, anus, genitals, and perineum (the external region between the genitals and the anus). The ring muscles are located at the ends of the important organ systems, like the alimentary, respiratory, and urogenital tracts. For the body to be in optimal health, it is very important that all the ring muscles contract simultaneously, establishing the inner rhythm and structure of the body.

The Taoists discovered the secrets of the ring muscles by observing infants and children. One of the goals of Taoist practice

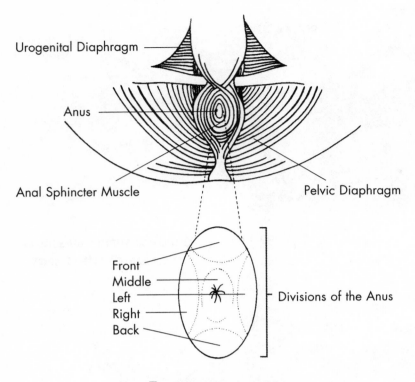

Urogenital Diaphragm

Anus

Anal Sphincter Muscle

Pelvic Diaphragm

Front
Middle
Left
Right
Back

Divisions of the Anus

THE ANAL RING MUSCLE

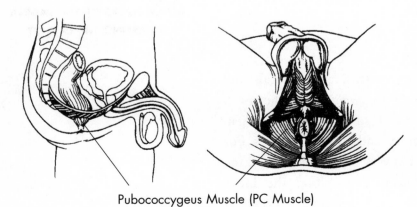

Pubococcygeus Muscle (PC Muscle)

PUBOCOCCYGEUS, OR PC, MUSCLE

is to become as vibrant and youthful as a child. Through specific exercises, the ring muscles bring our bodies back into harmony with the Tao.

Observe a newborn nursing: As the mouth rhythmically suckles, the eyes contract in unison, the anus and urinary tract contract and release in harmony with the mouth, and the hands open and close synchronistically with the sucking of the mouth. This synchronized movement pumps energy throughout the body.

Accordingly, when we as adults have a harmonious contraction and relaxation of the ring muscles, the body is full of energy and in good health. In contrast, when this rhythm is out of balance, from stress, sickness, or tension, the body's energy is depleted.

All the ring muscles in the body reflect one another. Sexual reflexology reveals this intimate connection among all the ring muscles in the body. The ring muscles in the face reveal the ring muscles in the urogenital tract, the anus, and the perineum. When there is an imbalance of sexual energy, it is revealed in the external characteristics of the face; for example, one eye or one side of the mouth may droop.

Also, the ring muscles directly influence the health of the internal organs. When the ring muscles are out of balance, the organs become depleted. This depletion in the organs is reflected to the sexual center, as the organs supply the sexual center with energy. All these internal dynamics are reflected in the face, hands, hair, and general external characteristics of the body. When the ring muscles are in balance, the hair will be shiny and healthy, and the skin clear and glowing.

The following series of exercises is designed to enhance the body's sphincter muscles.

EXERCISING THE RING MUSCLES

Contract the Mouth ◈ Suck the cheeks into the mouth, creating a suction in the mouth. It is very similar to the sensation of making "fish lips." Contract and relax at least nine to thirty-six times. Feel the connection between the mouth and the rest of the body. Notice the connection between the mouth and the lower ring muscles in the anus and perineum (which men feel at the base of the penis and women feel in the lower part of the vagina).

Blink the Eyes ◈ Rapidly blink the eyes and look around the room. Exercising the ring muscles around the eyes will improve vision and keep the eyes moist. It is also a very good exercise to wake the body up, as it stimulates the nerves. Blink the eyes for at least thirty seconds to one minute. Stimulating the muscles around the eyes helps open the urogenital diaphragm.

Contract the Anus ◈ Contract and relax the anus. Feel the energy from the lower centers surge through the body. There are many Taoist exercises that utilize the power of the anus to circulate energy. The Taoists believe that the strength of the anus is an indispensable aspect of overall health. By contracting the anus, we strengthen the connection to all the ring muscles in the body.

Contract the Perineum and Vagina ◈ Contract and release the muscles in the perineum and vagina. You are using a huge band of muscle—the pubococcygeus, or PC muscle— that is connected to the pubic and coccyx bones, the same muscle that is used to stop the flow of urination. This muscle, like the anus, is the floor of the sexual center. By strengthening the perineum and vagina, we are able to contain sexual energy rather than allowing it to drain out of the body. Developing the strength of the perineum is the first step in many other Taoist practices. You can contract and relax the perineum, vagina, and anus at the same time to create more power in the urogenital diaphragm.

Full Body Contraction   ◆   Contract and relax all the ring muscles simultaneously. Contract the eyes shut, suck in the mouth, squeeze the anus, and pull up on the perineum all at once. Then relax. Do this at least nine to thirty-six times. This will greatly strengthen the whole body. Remember that when all the ring muscles are in harmony, the body is vibrant and full of life force.

Contracting the eyes, mouth, anus, and perineum will activate the center of the brain. When you contract the perineum, the PC muscle squeezes the prostate gland, activating the pineal gland, to which it is closely connected. The pineal gland is regarded as the second sexual organ.

MALE PELVIC VISCERA, PROSTATE, BASE OF THE PENIS, AND PERINEUM

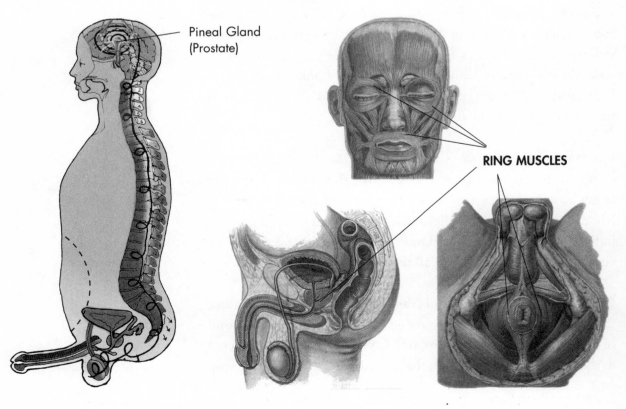

Pineal Gland
(Prostate)

RING MUSCLES

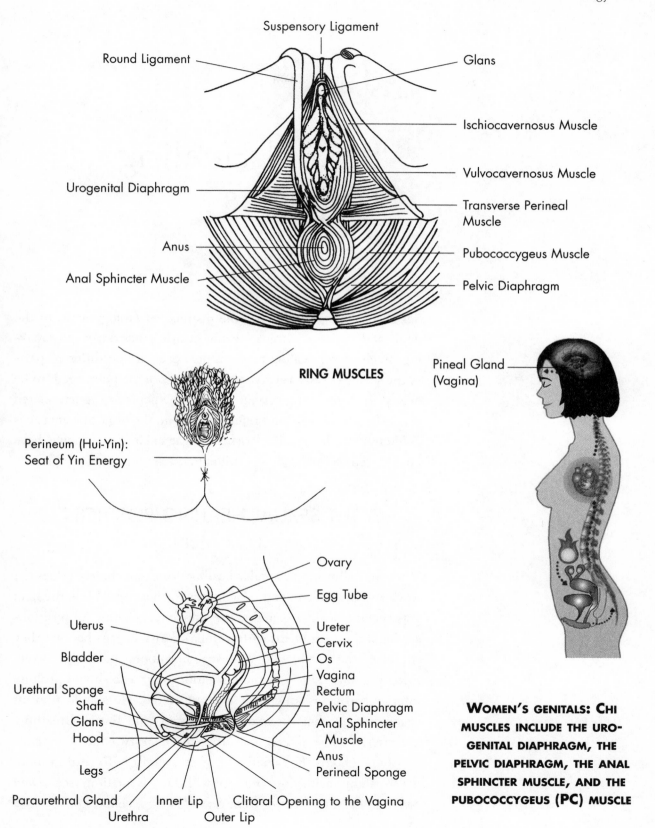

Suspensory Ligament

Round Ligament

Glans

Ischiocavernosus Muscle

Vulvocavernosus Muscle

Urogenital Diaphragm

Transverse Perineal Muscle

Anus

Pubococcygeus Muscle

Anal Sphincter Muscle

Pelvic Diaphragm

RING MUSCLES

Pineal Gland (Vagina)

Perineum (Hui-Yin): Seat of Yin Energy

Ovary

Egg Tube

Uterus

Ureter

Cervix

Bladder

Os

Vagina

Urethral Sponge

Rectum

Shaft

Pelvic Diaphragm

Glans

Anal Sphincter Muscle

Hood

Anus

Legs

Perineal Sponge

Paraurethral Gland   Inner Lip   Clitoral Opening to the Vagina

Urethra   Outer Lip

WOMEN'S GENITALS: CHI MUSCLES INCLUDE THE URO-GENITAL DIAPHRAGM, THE PELVIC DIAPHRAGM, THE ANAL SPHINCTER MUSCLE, AND THE PUBOCOCCYGEUS (PC) MUSCLE

Sexual Healing Positions

Sexual healing positions use the distinct reflexology areas of the penis and vagina to target specific health issues during lovemaking. Each sexual healing position puts pressure on different parts of the sexual organs, relative to which part of the body needs to be healed. In stimulating certain areas of the penis or vagina, related organs are stimulated and rejuvenated, and the orgasmic energy is guided up to the specific organs. These ancient techniques have been tested and proven over millennia.

EIGHT SEXUAL HEALING POSITIONS FOR MEN

With the following particular healing positions, the man does the work and the woman is the facilitator for healing. While the man gets specific healing benefits, the woman also gains. All positions are helpful for problems with women's sexual organs because they stimulate the production of sexual hormones and help correct menstrual difficulties. In these positions the male should prolong intercourse for as long as it is comfortable. He should prevent ejaculation by using the anal contractions of the Testicle Breathing exercises. (Taoist intercourse using ejaculatory control tremendously heightens the benefits of these exercises. To read in more depth about achieving orgasm without ejaculation, see *Taoist Secrets of Love: Cultivating Male Sexual Energy*, chapter 8.

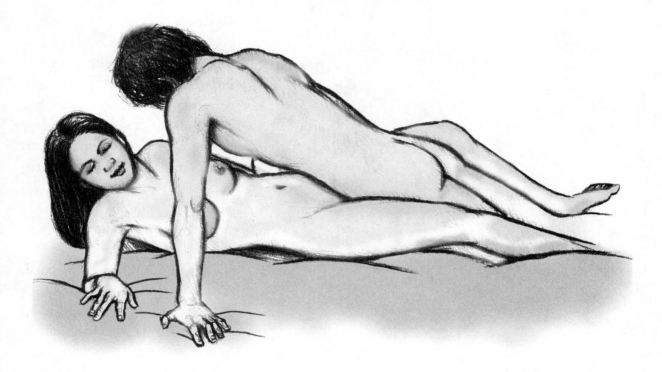

POSITION 1: ASSISTS IN SEX-RELATED PROBLEMS SUCH AS IMPOTENCE, PREMATURE EJACULATION, AND DIFFICULTY IN ACHIEVING ORGASM

Position 1 ◈ The woman reclines on her side with her hips rotated so that her pelvis faces upward. The man is above and enters her with his penis. This improves all sex-related problems, including impotence. Nearly all men have some sexual ability, and thus it is quite uncommon to be totally impotent. Most of the time in instances of impotency the erection is lost about halfway into the vagina or sometime during intercourse. Failure to reach a climax often occurs because the man is not being totally present. His mind roams and he drifts off into some fantasy. Because this position is a bit clumsy for the man, he must concentrate on what he is doing. Consequently, his mind will not wander or fantasize. At first, just relax and focus on inserting the penis, then do whatever comes naturally to you, at your own pace. It may take some time to gain self-confidence.

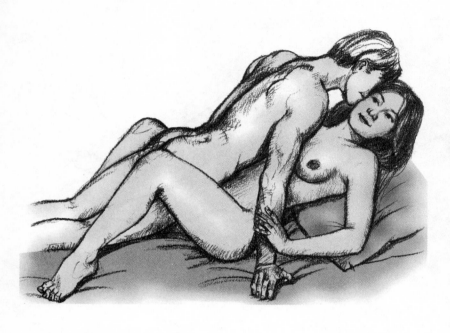

POSITION 2: ENERGIZES THE BODY

POSITION 3: STRENGTHENS INTERNAL ORGANS,
INCLUDING THE KIDNEYS, SPLEEN, AND LIVER

Position 2 ◈ The woman reclines on her back. She supports her head and shoulders with a large, high pillow. Then she bends forward at the neck. In such a position the vagina is slightly curved, which allows the penis to be massaged in the right location. Entering from the front, the man penetrates with his penis. After making love in this position every day for two or three days, the body will be totally rejuvenated. There are benefits for the woman as well because air is drawn up into the vagina, which stimulates her internal organs.

Position 3 ◈ Both individuals lie on their sides face-to-face. The woman keeps her lower leg straight and bends her upper leg backward. The man inserts his penis. Make love in this position for a maximum of four times a day for twenty days.

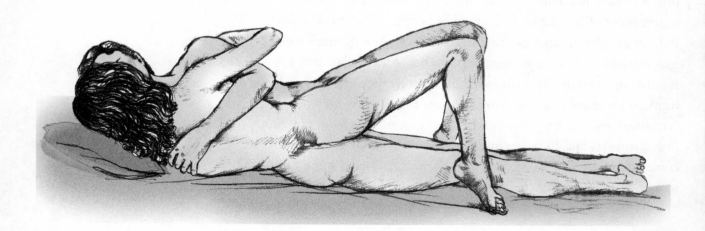

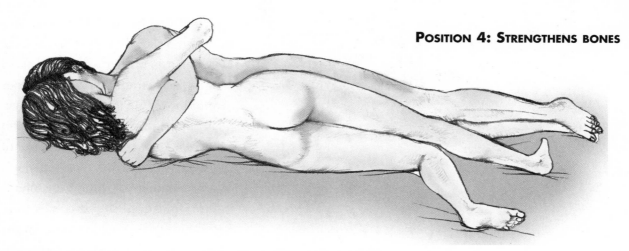

POSITION 4: STRENGTHENS BONES

Position 4 ◈ The woman reclines on her left side. She bends her left leg as far as possible toward her back. The right leg remains straight. Face-to-face with her, the man finds an angle where he can enter her vagina. He can be a bit on top of her or immediately face-to-face. Use this position for a maximum of five times a day over a ten-day period. This is excellent for healing arthritis, leukemia, and bone marrow diseases. Furthermore, it can speed up healing of broken bones.

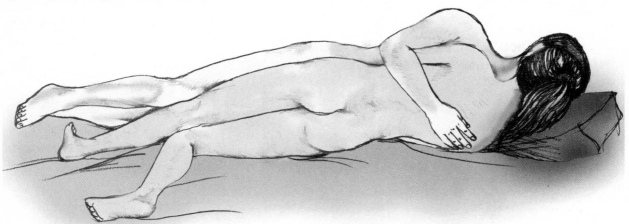

POSITION 5: ASSISTS BLOOD VESSEL PROBLEMS

Position 5 ◈ This position is similar to position 4 except the woman reclines on her right side with her right leg bent. The man enters her the same way, face-to-face but a little bit above. Work in this position a maximum of six times a day for twenty days. This approach is good for all sorts of blood vessel difficulties, including varicose veins and hardening of the arteries. It also improves high or low blood pressure.

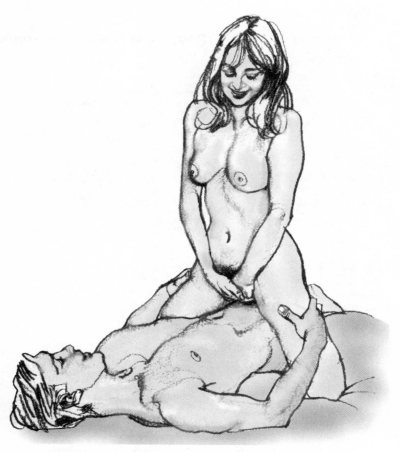

Position 6 ✦ The man lies down relaxed on his back. The woman is on her knees and faces him. He enters her but she does not move. He moves up and down from beneath her. This position can be used for a maximum of seven times a day for ten days. All manner of blood problems are improved by this position, including anemia, low blood pressure, poor blood quality, and blood clots.

POSITION 6: ADDRESSES BLOOD PROBLEMS, INCLUDING BLOOD PRESSURE

Position 7 ✦ The man lies relaxed on his back. The woman kneels above him on her hands and knees. She faces him and can move a little. Essentially, though, only the man moves after penetration. Use this position a maximum of eight times a day for about fifteen days.

POSITION 7: ASSISTS LYMPHATIC SYSTEM PROBLEMS

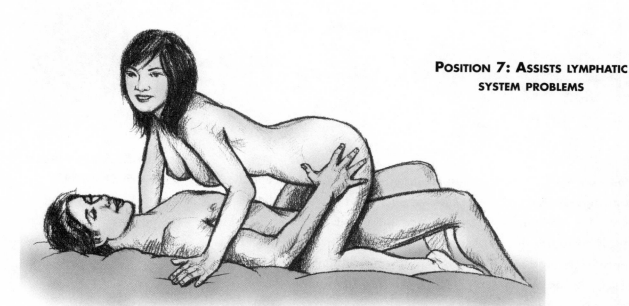

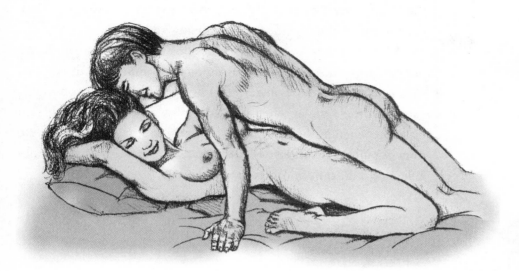

Position 8 ◈ This position is often hard for the woman. She gets on her knees and then bends all the way backward with her feet under her. She bends back until her head and back are on the bed. The man enters her from in front and above. The woman may want to put a pillow behind her. Use this position a maximum of nine times a day for ten days.

When the woman is in this position, the shape of the vagina is changed. The friction from the man's thrusting affects different areas of the penis. Through the process of reflexology, this influences different parts of the body and provides healing stimulation. The male heals himself and the woman is the facilitator. In the woman's healing positions that follow, the woman heals herself and the man is the facilitator.

SEVEN SEXUAL HEALING POSITIONS FOR WOMEN

With the following positions the male works for the woman. However, unlike the benefits the woman gets from the male's healing positions, he receives no real healing benefit.

How deeply the penis penetrates is important in the woman's healing positions. This is because different reflexology zones are located along the length of the vagina. Thus, different portions of the vagina need massage. Penetration can be shallow or deep, depending on the specific problem being addressed.

After the penis is inserted in these positions, the woman moves her pelvis for the purpose of massaging and stimulating the vagina. When necessary, the man restrains himself and should communicate with the woman when he has to slow down. He should not ejaculate when in these positions. Repetition requirements are the same for all the positions: They may be done as many as nine times a day for a maximum of ten days.

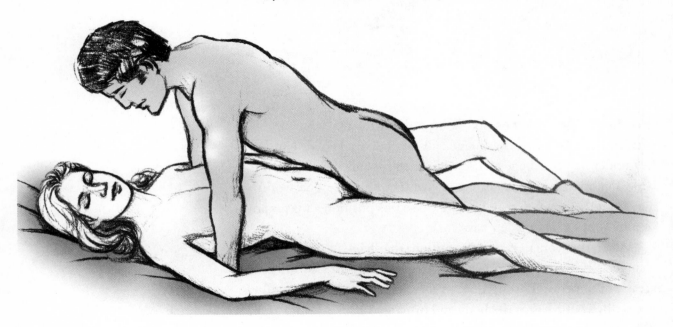

POSITION 1: FOR FATIGUE AS EVIDENCED BY BLURRY VISION, HEAVY PERSPIRATION, WEAKNESS, FAINTING, QUICK HEARTBEAT, AND WEAK, SHALLOW, AND RAPID BREATHING

Position 1 ❖ The woman lies flat on her back and the man is on top of her. He inserts his penis as deeply as he can. The woman rotates in a circular motion beneath him, moving clockwise as well as counterclockwise. The man allows the woman to work and stays in this position until she is satisfied. Orgasm is not, however, the object of the healing exercises, and healing benefits will occur even without orgasm.

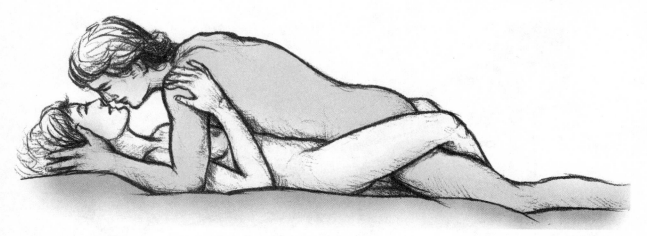

Position 2 ◈ The woman reclines on her back and wraps her legs around the man's thighs but not his back or shoulders. The man is above her on his hands and knees and inserts the head of his penis only about one and one-half to two inches. As in position 1, the woman circles in both directions for as long as she feels comfortable. Because the man is on his hands and knees, there is shallow penetration. This means that the penis touches only the lung, pancreas, and heart reflexology zones of the vagina. This position is also good for all the joints.

POSITION 2: STIMULATES THE PANCREAS AND LIVER, IS HELPFUL FOR DIABETICS; ALSO AIDS WITH HOT FLASHES, WEAK KNEES, AND SORE FEET AND KNEES AFTER STANDING FOR A LONG TIME

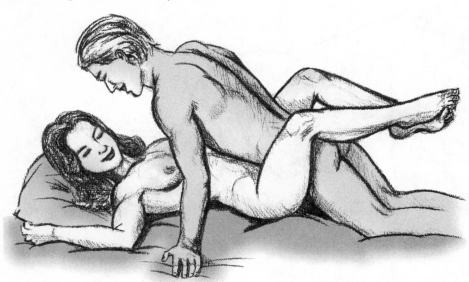

Position 3 ◈ The woman reclines on her back with her legs locked around the man's midsection. She wraps her arms around him. On his hands and knees, he penetrates her halfway. Once again the woman rotates in one direction and then the other for as long as she is comfortable.

POSITION 3: ASSISTS THE STOMACH, SPLEEN, AND FEMALE ORGANS AND AIDS DIGESTIVE PROBLEMS

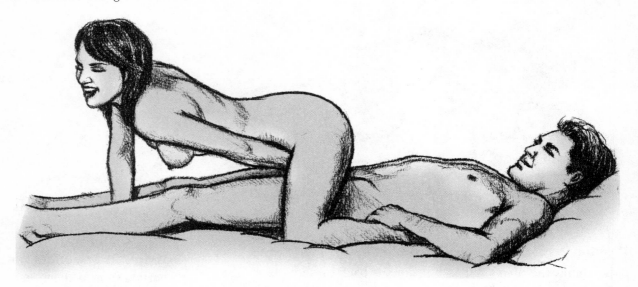

POSITION 4: HELPS WITH WATER RETENTION, KIDNEY AND BLADDER AILMENTS, CHRONIC HIGH FEVER, AND PITUITARY GLAND PROBLEMS

Position 4 ◈ The man lies on his back. The woman is on her knees facing the man's feet. The man inserts only the head of his penis. The woman can hold the penis for better control. As in the previous positions, she circles in both directions as long as she feels comfortable.

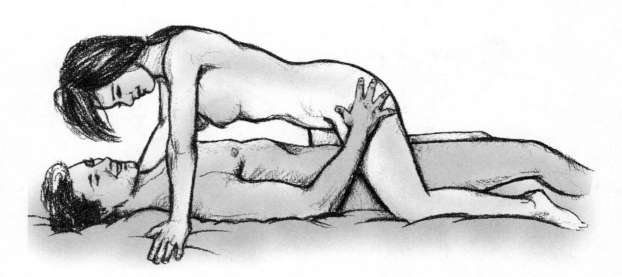

POSITION 5: ASSISTS WITH THE NERVOUS SYSTEM, LIVER, ULCERS, AND EYESIGHT

Position 5 ◈ The man lies on his back, with the woman on her knees facing him. The penetration of the vagina alternates from shallow to deep as the woman moves up and down on the penis. As she does so, she also rotates her pelvis. This gives the vagina a complete massage.

Nervous system problems trouble many women. The female menstrual cycle can lead to hormonal imbalances and impact the nervous system. Childbearing can add to the hormonal imbalances that some women experience. This is a very good position to help bring the woman's nervous system into balance.

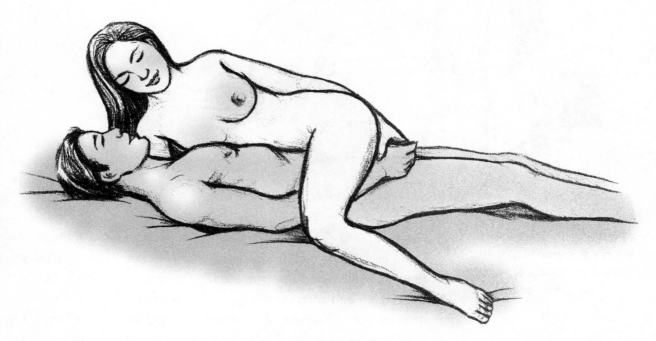

Position 6 ❖ The man lies relaxed on his back and the woman is on her knees, supporting herself with one elbow. She is just a little to the side of the man. She holds his penis. With her other hand she holds his head. The penis is allowed to penetrate halfway, but she holds it the entire time. Once again, she rotates in this position for as long as she is comfortable. (Penetration in this position is not easy. That is why the woman must hold the penis.)

POSITION 6: ADDRESSES ENERGY BLOCKAGES IN THE MERIDIANS, HEADACHES, POOR CIRCULATION, MENSTRUAL PROBLEMS

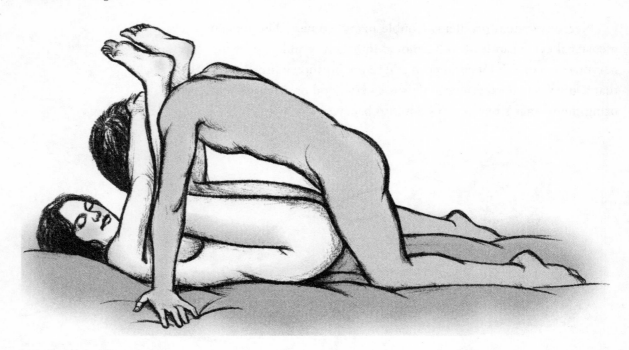

POSITION 7: HELPS WITH BLOOD SHORTAGE, ANEMIA, POOR CIRCULATION, AND PALE, DRY SKIN

Position 7 ◈ This position is not as difficult as some of the others. The woman reclines on her back. Her knees are up to her chest and her feet are in the air. The man rests on his knees in front of her and enters very deeply. The woman rotates as the man remains still. This position contracts the vagina, which allows for very deep penetration. If the man has a very long penis, he can wrap the base of the shaft with a handkerchief to prevent it from going too far into the vagina. (This should always be done if the penis is longer than the partner's vagina.) In addition, the handkerchief makes the penis stand up more and helps preserve the erection. The principle is the same as a "cock ring," which blocks the blood vessels so the blood cannot flow back out of the penis as easily.

EXCHANGE OF ENERGY AS A SEXUAL HEALING PRAYER

What is true love? Love combined with truth equals true love. While the word *love* has different meanings, *true love* means that two hearts are united and there is no gap between them. It is not a social love. The love for a wife or husband is different from the love for a friend. Even the closest friends have a gap between them.

Neither gender should live alone. This is not meant in the sense of actually sharing living quarters but from the point of view of sexual relationships. The sexes need each other for gratification and in order to heal, balance, and adjust their physical bodies. We know from Taoism that every part of the body is holy.

In order to have a full life as human beings, we need to understand our sexuality. To do so is to have a divine life. Suffering is not divine. When people reach a certain level of existence, they become spiritual. The notion of suffering to become spiritual is actually an ego-bound concept. People are not forced to suffer. We have a choice. If people had no willpower or choice, they would be machines. If we are to please God, we must please ourselves first, because God is in us. If we lead a divine life, we are already in God's kingdom. There is no need to pay a duty to God. He is capable of doing whatever he needs for himself.

It is the goal of the Tao to become one complete person. Male and female can be united and become one complete person through what is known as Sexual Healing Prayers, a form of meditation allowing a couple to connect with divine energy while in sexual union. Sexual Healing Prayers involve the exchange of energy during orgasm with intention of healing for both lovers. A lot of discipline is required of the man during Sexual Healing Prayers. This helps prevent him from giving in to lust. The man attends to the woman with his body. Sexual Healing Prayers allow people to start and end the day in peace away from worries and struggles.

Because we have our bodies, we should use them and discipline them. They are an instrument for the soul-mind to follow the spirit. If we allow our spirit to lead us and we follow our intuition, our conscience, and communication with God, our thinking, emotions, and decisions come along too. It is, of course, impossible to get rid of our bodies. They must be satisfied. Sexual Healing Prayers both satisfy and discipline the body at the same time. When we pray, we should request that our bodies listen to our spirit. We decide to please our God-self. We will have a feeling of pure love.

As soon as two people meet, they become comparable to a square. Throughout the Sexual Healing Prayers they are interlaced and share a meeting point, at which time the square turns into a triangle. The woman is totally open and receiving. She is completely yin. The male is at his Taoist orgasm (orgasm without ejaculation) and is giving completely. He is completely yang. The complete yin state and complete yang state make up a perfect yin-yang balance, which becomes a circle that has no beginning and no end. There are no cracks and no sharpness in the circle, since there is no criticism between the man and the woman. For the partners there is only feeling, devoid of judgment or thinking. With their eyes closed they feel each other. This feeling is total love and perfect unification. This union comprises the yin-yang. It is the microcosm and the macrocosm of the universe. It is eternal.

At that instant the partners are beyond space and time. Even if the prayer takes only two minutes, that in itself is time without end. The woman's climax during the Sexual Healing Prayer may last from two to ten or twenty minutes. During that period she is totally at ease and has no other physical desire. Consequently, the Sexual Healing Prayer is a kind of meditation. The quivering body and vaginal fluids are a part of the climax and may happen a few times before the woman is entirely opened up. The Sexual Healing Prayer for the man is the point just before ejaculation, but when he gets to that stage he remains there and holds it, using only feeling and no knowledge. Indeed, this is the Tree of Life. More than an erection is required for Sexual Healing Prayer. The prostate gland must be swollen to around 98 percent in order to keep the man's interest up.

Sometimes the purpose of meditation is misunderstood and it is often mixed up with "thinking." Many times when facing a problem people say, "I'll have to meditate on it." The meaning here is "to think." However, the real aim of meditation is to connect with our God-self.

Sexual Healing Prayers are the finest meditation possible. They blend communication with our God-self with inner exercise and healing. This is the level of absolute unity, or "no mind." Once this level is reached, people find themselves so fulfilled that they have no desire left for ordinary human sex. Love is beyond studying or teaching. Its origin is the heart, and it is genuinely spiritual from the beginning. Love is giving.

During the Sexual Healing Prayer the man gives himself to his lover. The woman's gift lies in her surrender to the man. The two grow together, trading energy and well-being. Thus, sex can be used by people to feel divinity. The Sexual Healing Prayers provide total love automatically. This is not, however, the same as the mental picture of romantic love that most people have in their minds. It can be said that it is the apogee of Taoist sexology. Just as the day is started with the morning Sexual Healing Prayer, so too is it concluded with the evening Sexual Healing Prayer. The experience is delightful. People find that they go to sleep relaxed and peaceful. The next day when they wake up they are prepared for the morning Sexual Healing Prayer.

We must realize that our thoughts form our world. The mind's cognition is essential reality and it comes long before the material world. The material things we can touch and see are brought into existence by the mind. With the right thoughts, anything can be materialized. Thus, in this case, we need merely to concentrate on the right partner and visualize what we want in our mind. Doing this will create the right person for us.

5

Sexual Energizing Postures

One of the core principles of the Healing Love practices is that the Taoists do not differentiate between sex and body, using one word—jing—to describe both. Using your hands to touch, stimulate and bring your partner's attention and energy to various parts of the body, orients the lovemaking to the whole body instead of just a genital focus.

HAND POSITIONS

These are the basic hand positions for energizing the body and drawing the sexual energy into the brain while doing the Healing Love practices.

Using these hand positions during resting periods when making love draws the energy to the brain, enlarging the sexual organs and the size of the brain and pineal gland, giving you strength in the mind (brain) and body (organs). Each partner takes turns giving and receiving this gentle touch, while both partners focus on internal meditation.

SACRAL PUMP ENERGY POINT

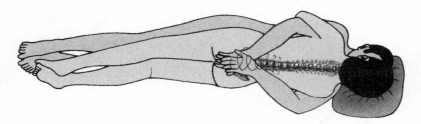

Position 1 ❖ This hand position strengthens the semen and ovaries, activating the sacral pump.

Position 2 ◈ This hand position strengthens the life force and bone marrow, activating the *ming-men* point.

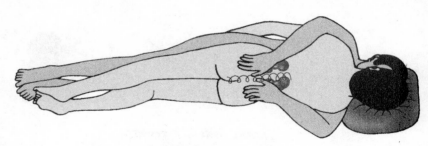

KIDNEYS ENERGY POINT

Position 3 ◈ This hand position strengthens all the organs and creates more sexual appeal, activating the Door of Life.

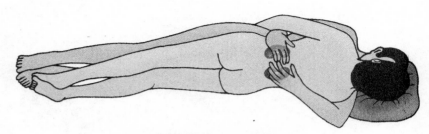

ADRENAL GLANDS POINT

Position 4 ◈ This hand position strengthens the bones and enhances face, eyes, and mouth color for a healthier, brighter-looking facial appearance, activating the T-11 (thoracic vertebra no. 11) point.

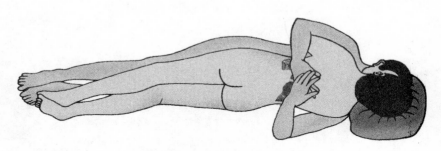

LIVER AND SPLEEN POINT

Position 5 ◈ This hand position strengthens the aorta and vena cava arteries, increasing the penis hardness and vaginal wetness, activating the wing point.

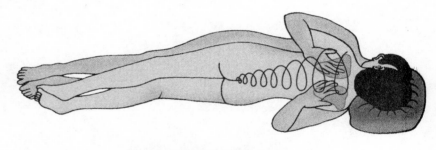

HEART AND LUNGS POINT

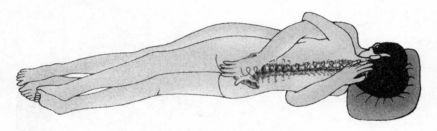

SACRAL AND C-7 POINTS

Position 6 ◈ This hand position strengthens the liver and spleen, creating sexy eyes and a sexier mouth, activating the C-7 point.

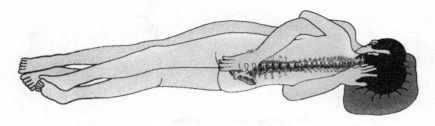

SACRAL AND NECK POINTS

Position 7 ◈ This hand position strengthens all the bones and improves the blood flow to the sexual organs, activating the sacral and cranial pumps.

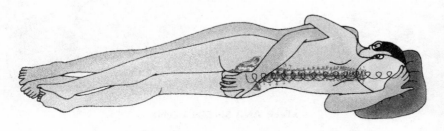

SACRAL AND CROWN POINTS

Position 8 ◈ This hand position strengthens the white and red blood cells and improves penile erection and vaginal wetness, opening up women to a greater orgasm by activating the crown point.

USE EYE MOVEMENTS IN HEALING LOVE POSTURES

The following illustrations show how to move your eyes to energize the senses. Energy will follow the movement of the eyes. Eye movement circulates and helps to collect the energy generated by the healing love session. Relax as you move the eyes, visualizing and allowing the sexual energy to flow where you direct your eyes inside your body. For example, if your eyes are to the left, allow the sexual energy to flow to the left side of the body.

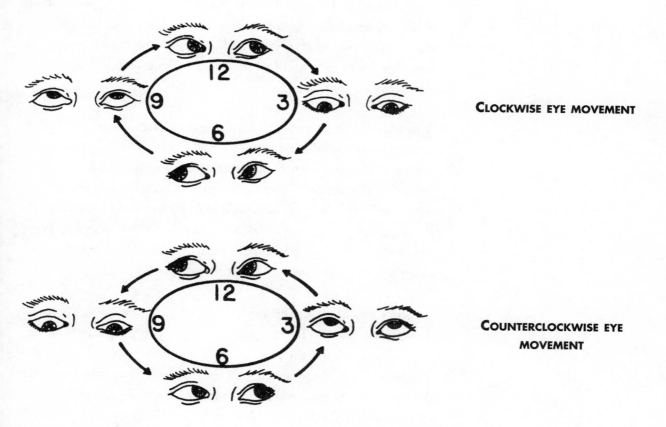

CLOCKWISE EYE MOVEMENT

COUNTERCLOCKWISE EYE MOVEMENT

Use mind and eyes to help circulate the energy nine times clockwise and nine times counterclockwise and collect the energy.

HEALING LOVE COUPLES
ENERGIZE THE SENSES

The Chi generated in the Healing Love can be circulated and sent to move into different parts of the body. The Chi collected in this way is very healing and powerful.

Improve the eyes ❖ When you are experiencing a high level of sexual energy and are near ejaculation, exhale through the mouth. Hold the breath, open the eyes wide and look left and right. Inhale and suck in the lower abdomen, then exhale relaxing the abdomen outward, six times. (This is called reverse breathing, because it is the reverse of what we normally do.) Balance the breath by breathing normally, and feel the orgasmic energy flow into all the meridians.

Improve the hearing ❖ When close to ejaculation and experiencing a high level of orgasmic sexual energy, swallow the saliva, which is charged with Chi, down to the Lower Tan Tien (navel center) six times and grind your teeth with closed mouth. Inhale, hold the breath for a while, and listen to the sound inside the ears. Exhale, flatten the stomach. Inhale, suck up the stomach, hold, and let the orgasmic Chi spread to the limbs and the whole body. This will improve the hearing until old age.

Balance organs ❖ This exercise improves digestion and cures all kinds of diseases. When the sexual energy is very high and ejaculation is near, expand the stomach and use mind power to gather the orgasmic Chi in the stomach. Contract the perineum and anus. This will help the orgasm circulate to all the body organs and glands. After this, do the Nine Shallow and One Deep thrusting pattern. The movement of the penis in and out of the vagina should be in a screwing fashion (that is how the slang expression originated) going clockwise in and counterclockwise out. The ancient expression of "don't stab the lady" refers to this. This will help gather the orgasmic Chi; negative Chi will disperse.

Strengthen erection ❖ Practice the headstand to help reverse the sexual energy to the head and to all the body. This will make the penis hard, with a strong erection. After lovemaking is a particularly good time to do this, as most circulation happens during the resting period of the healing love. Hold the headstand just for a few minutes, or as long as you can. Return the Chi and balance the yin and yang: When close to ejaculation, inhale nine times, hold back the ejaculation (with mind power). Use the left hand to hold the testicles, and feel the orgasmic Chi turn to sexual fluid.

Semen retention: Those who release semen only twice monthly, or twenty-four times a year, have more potential to live to one or two hundred years, with fine complexions and no ailments. Chapter 6 provides instruction in ejaculation control.

HEALING LOVE POSTURES FOR UNIVERSAL TAO PRACTICES

The sitting position is perfect for later lovemaking and energy connection and circulation for Microcosmic Orbit meditation.

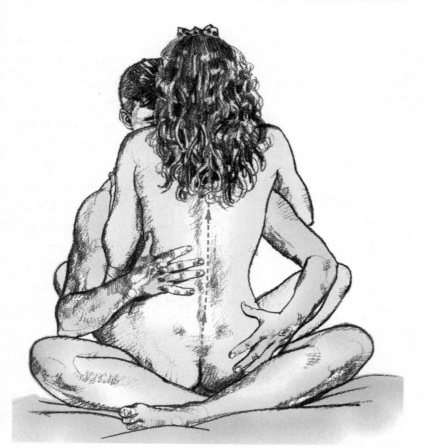

MICROCOSMIC ORBIT CONNECTION

CIRCULATING SEXUAL ENERGY IN MICROCOSMIC ORBIT

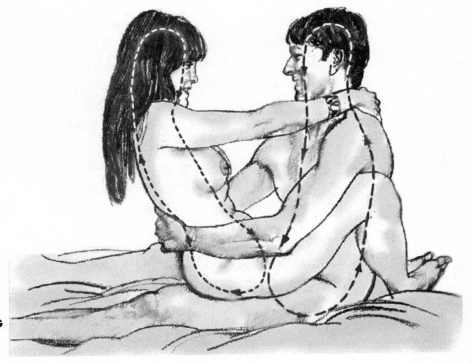

EXCHANGING AND MOVING THE HEALING SEXUAL ENERGY ON THE MICROCOSMIC ORBIT

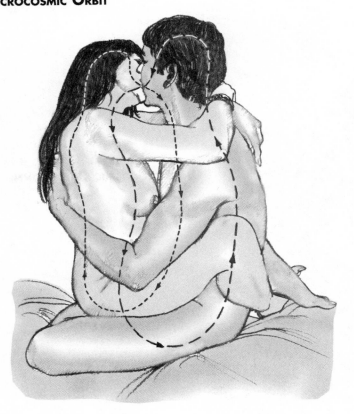

Couples must first learn to circulate sexual energy in their own bodies during lovemaking. Later, partners can learn to give and receive sexual energy by using the Microcosmic Orbit.

Exchanging and moving the energy allows the couples to give and receive sexual energy fully in healing each other through the Microcosmic Orbit meditation.

ENERGIZING POSTURES WITH EIGHT HEALING BENEFITS

Practice the Microcosmic Orbit in all of the following postures. To strengthen the organs and senses, you can use the sexual energy by stimulating the sexual reflexology points. The organs and senses become stronger and you become more attractive and sexier.

Position 1 ◈ The first benefit, "to firm up the semen," is achieved by carrying out a count of double nine (eighteen) penetrations. Rest and use the Microcosmic Orbit to guide the orgasmic Chi up to the crown. Do this twice. When the count is completed, the man stops; this causes him to make the semen healthy. To eliminate blood leakage between periods, the woman should practice twice daily and she should be fine in fifteen days.

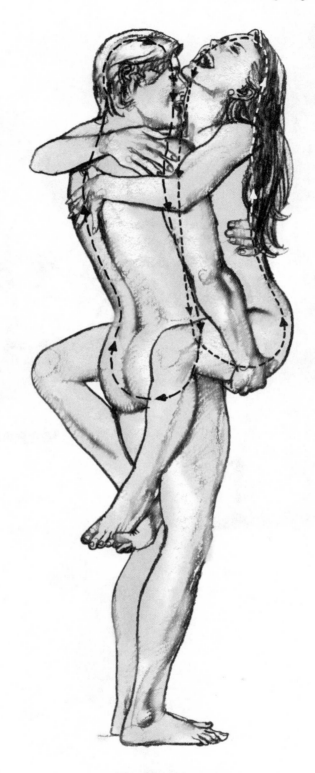

FIRMING UP SEMEN

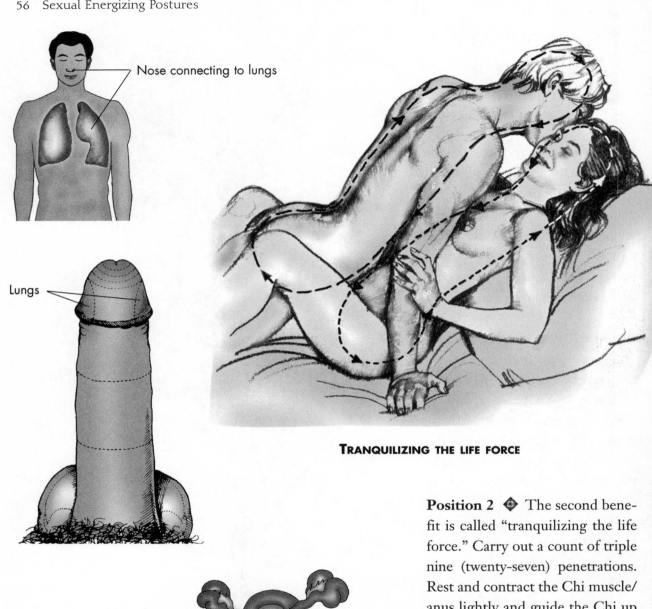

Nose connecting to lungs

Lungs

TRANQUILIZING THE LIFE FORCE

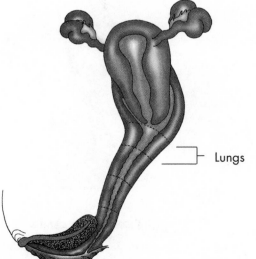

Lungs

Position 2 ✦ The second benefit is called "tranquilizing the life force." Carry out a count of triple nine (twenty-seven) penetrations. Rest and contract the Chi muscle/anus lightly and guide the Chi up to the lungs; do this exercise three more times in succession for the life force to be harmonized.

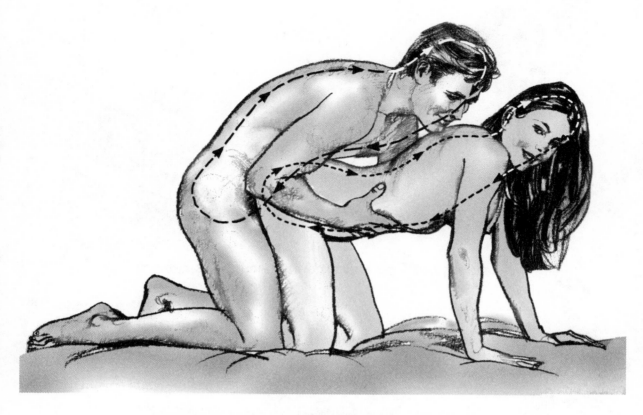

PROFITABLY HOARDING: STRENGTHENING ALL THE SENSES

Position 3 ◈ The third benefit is called "profitably hoarding." Carry out a count of four nines (thirty-six) penetrations and stop when the count is completed. Rest and guide Chi into the organs; do four sets. This causes the couple's life force to be harmonized; it can help coolness of the woman's gate (vagina).

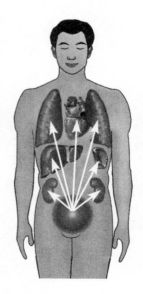

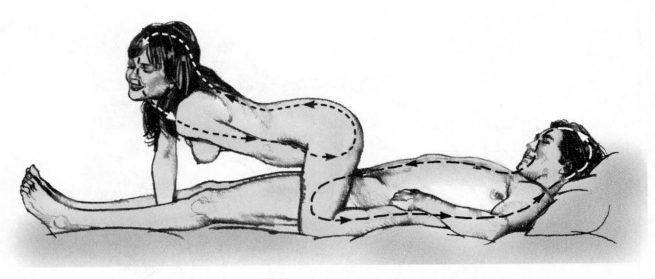

STRENGTHENING THE BONES: CONNECTING KIDNEYS AND EYES

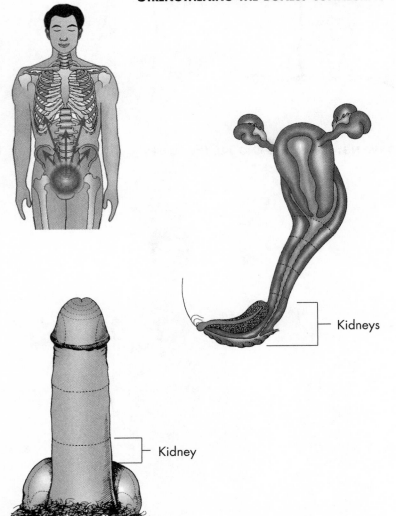

Kidneys

Kidney

Position 4 ❖ The fourth bene-fit is "strengthening the bones." Carry out a count of five nines (forty-five) penetrations and stop when the count is completed. Rest and guide orgasmic Chi into the bones of the spine and rib cage and the hip bones. Do five sets. In Chinese medicine the kidneys are said to rule the bones, because the bone marrow makes the blood and the kidneys filter the blood. This position stimulates the kid-neys, while the eyes are used to move the Chi around in the orbit and to the bones. This causes an improvement of the articulation of the joints in the man allowing more flexibility and strength; it can remove obstruction of the woman's blood.

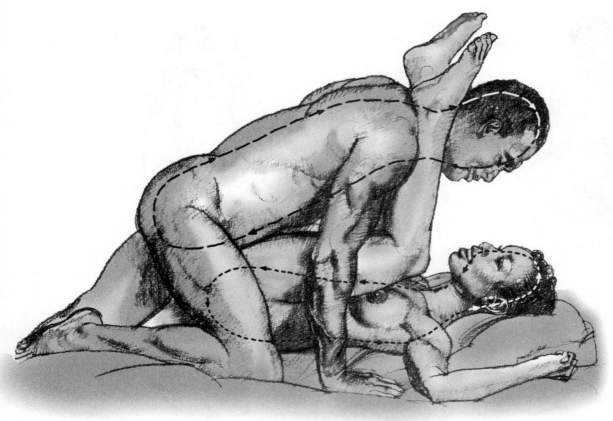

BLENDING THE CONDUITS

Position 5 ❖ The fifth benefit is "blending the conduits"; carry out a count of six nines (fifty-four) penetrations and stop when the count is completed. Rest and guide orgasmic Chi into the aorta and the vena cava. Do six sets.

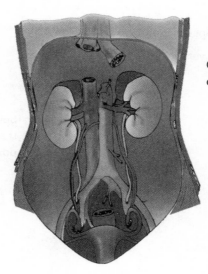

Guide chi into the aorta and vena cava

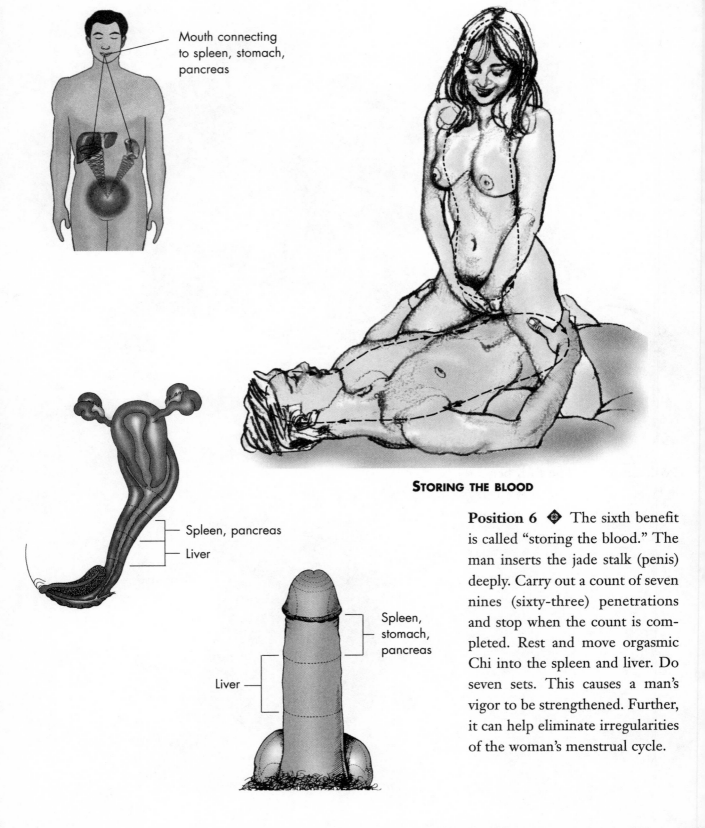

Mouth connecting
to spleen, stomach,
pancreas

Spleen, pancreas
Liver

Spleen,
stomach,
pancreas

Liver

STORING THE BLOOD

Position 6 ❖ The sixth benefit is called "storing the blood." The man inserts the jade stalk (penis) deeply. Carry out a count of seven nines (sixty-three) penetrations and stop when the count is completed. Rest and move orgasmic Chi into the spleen and liver. Do seven sets. This causes a man's vigor to be strengthened. Further, it can help eliminate irregularities of the woman's menstrual cycle.

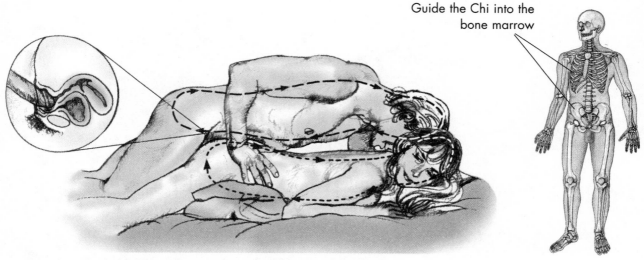

Guide the Chi into the bone marrow

PROFITING THE FLUID: CONNECTING KIDNEYS AND EYES

Position 7 ◈ The seventh benefit is "profiting the fluid." The man mounts the woman, carries out a count of eight nines (seventy-two) penetrations, and stops when the count is completed. Rest. With the eyes, guide the orgasmic Chi into the bone marrow in the hips and rib cage. Do eight sets.

INFORMING THE BODY: EXPANDING THE CHI INTO THE BONES AND BONE MARROW

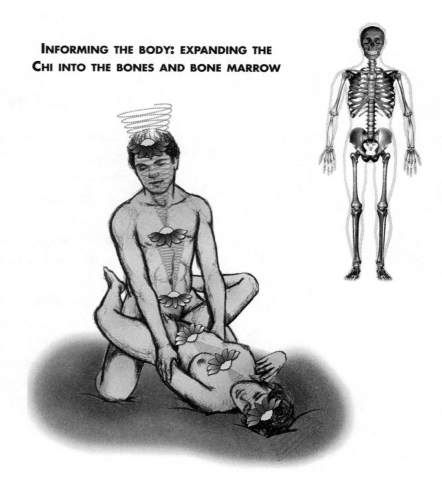

Position 8 ◈ The eighth benefit is "informing the body." The man carries out a count of nine nines (eighty-one) penetrations and stops when the count is completed. Rest and guide orgasmic Chi into the bones and bone marrow. Do nine sets. This practice causes the man's bones to be filled with Chi.

Ejaculation and Menstrual Management

A man may attain health and longevity if he practices an ejaculation frequency of twice monthly, or twenty-four times in a year. If at the same time he pays careful attention to proper diet and exercise, he will live a long and healthy life.

—Dr. Sun Ssu-mo

EJACULATION MANAGEMENT

Diet, exercise, and sexual restraint constitute the three pillars of Taoist health and longevity programs. Of course, these Taoist principles apply equally to males and females. For both genders, semen essence is the energy that propels sexuality. It is the origin of the physical ability for sex as well as sexual interest and emotional affection for the opposite sex. On the other hand, because women do not discharge when they reach orgasm, their sexual drive and interest are not diminished after one act of intercourse. Since the principles required to achieve the harmony of yin and yang should be cultivated mostly by men, much of this chapter is addressed mostly to them. However, the information in those sections should also be studied and comprehended by women who keep company with Taoist men or who wish to convert their men to Taoism (see *Taoist Secrets of Love* and *Healing Love through the Tao* by Mantak Chia). This chapter also includes a section devoted to cultivating women's sexual energy and strengthening women's sexual organs.

According to Western medicine, men naturally replace their semen soon after ejaculating and have a virtually limitless supply. This generalization is very misleading. Ejaculation can be compared to blood donation. After donating blood, people feel weak and tired for a day or two, until the lost blood is replenished. Blood clinics suggest that people donate only a few times each year in order to avoid chronic fatigue, lowered resistance, and excessive strain on the circulatory system. Chinese medicine holds that the same principle applies to semen, except that the lost semen is even more difficult to replace than blood. A great deal of essence and energy are needed to replace semen supplies completely and restore proper hormone balance after ejaculation.

If the frequency of ejaculation surpasses the body's ability to replace the semen completely, men go through chronic fatigue, decreased resistance, irritability, and other indications of depleted essence and energy. Furthermore, they lose all sexual interest in their partners, who could very well desire additional lovemaking. While it may be the case that adolescents and young men in their early twenties replace semen at a pace that permits frequent ejaculation, the idea that this ability goes on indefinitely into adulthood is absurd. Rather it is women, not men, whose sexual power is virtually unlimited. It should be noted, though, that celibacy is not the answer either, because that deprives men of the benefits of sexual stimulation. The solution, then, is ejaculation control. Regular coitus with infrequent ejaculation maintains a man's interest in the act and his ability to continue indefinitely until his mate is completely satisfied. In fact, males who ejaculate one or more times daily might eventually "lose their minds." Frequent ejaculation brings about a chronic loss of the vital fluid that the brain and spine need to operate properly. The resulting deficiency of this critical fluid may bring about premature senility, inability to concentrate, chronic depression, loss of sexual drive, and numerous related symptoms.

In addition, modern scientific evidence indicates that every time a man ejaculates, there is a meaningful loss of zinc. Zinc is a rare but extremely important trace element. Therefore, ejaculating

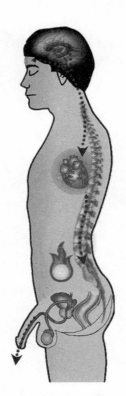

THROUGH EJACULATION ZINC IS LOST, WHICH LEADS TO LOSS OF MEMORY, CONFUSION, AND PARANOIA

too often results in a chronic and serious deficiency of zinc. The symptoms of zinc depletion include loss of memory, confusion, paranoia, and hypersensitivity to sunlight. It is interesting that these scientific facts seem to substantiate the "old wives' tale" that claimed that masturbating too often muddles the mind, weakens the spine, and causes blindness.

Regulating Ejaculation Frequency

Every school of Taoism believes that retaining semen and proper regulation are essential skills for men of the Way. The mavens of ancient China each left us their own personal guidelines determining emission frequency. By putting their different suggestions together with your personal requirements and actual experience, you can easily determine an ejaculation timetable that is appropriate for your personal needs.

To start, let's consider what the Plain Girl said to the Yellow Emperor on the topic. Being a bit confused by the notion of "sparing vital essence" and "regulating leakage," the Yellow Emperor expressed his doubts to the Plain Girl. This is what she had to say: Some men are strong, others weak. Some men are old, while others are young. Each person must live according to his own vital force and not try to impede the joys of sex. Impeding joy is harmful. The following is a list of the Plain Girl's recommendations.

1. A healthy male of twenty may ejaculate two times a day, but an old one should do so no more than once daily.

2. A thirty-year-old male can ejaculate once a day, but only once every two days if he is not strong.

3. A brandishing, vigorous forty-year-old man can give off semen once every three days, but if he is lacking power, he may do so only once every four days.

4. A full-bodied man fifty years old may eject semen once every five days, but only every ten days if he is lacking strength.

5. A healthy sixty-year-old man may ejaculate once every ten days, but only once every twenty days if he is in poor health.

6. A robust seventy-year-old man can eject semen once a month, but one lacking strength should no longer emit semen at all.

During the Tang dynasty, physician Lee Tung-hsuan, in *Mysterious Master of the Cave*, used the frequency of coitus, rather than the number of days, as his recommended measure for regulating emissions. For example, when having intercourse with women, a man should eject semen only two or three times in a ten-day period. The great Han dynasty adept Master Liu Ching, credited in dynastic archives with living more than three hundred years, preferred to regulate his semen ejection relative to the universal cycles of seasonal change.

The seasons have an influence on how often a man may allow himself to ejaculate. In spring, once every three days is reasonable, but in the summer and fall, twice a month is more appropriate. In the cold of winter, there should be no ejaculation at all. Accumulating yang essence in winter is the way of heaven. Those who follow this advice will live a long and healthy life. A single ejaculation in winter is one hundred times more harmful than a springtime ejaculation.

The best advice on the topic of ejaculation restraint comes from the centenarian doctor Sun Ssu-mo. This Tang dynasty Taoist outlived three emperors by following his own advice. The "twice-monthly" rule of thumb that he recommended is quoted at the beginning of this chapter. In actual practice, however, he ejaculated only one time per one hundred copulations. Dr. Sun lived to be 101.

Sun Ssu-mo tells us that a man should "become acquainted" with Taoism by the time he is thirty and "gain a complete working knowledge" of it by forty. Prior to the age of forty, most men are still extremely potent and vigorous. By the time he is forty, however, a man notices his potency decreasing. At the time that his potency

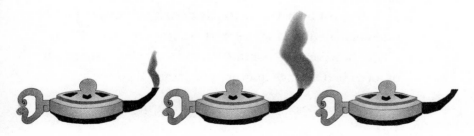

FIRE OF THE LAMPS

declines, numerous ailments will come upon him. Unchecked, he will quickly find himself beyond cure. Dr. Sun gives repeated warnings to his male patients of the dangers associated with excessive ejaculation. He makes an analogy with a sputtering oil lamp that, just prior to being spent, suddenly flares up brightly, then dies. Whenever a man restrains himself and holds on to his semen, it is like adding new oil to a lamp that is about to go out. But if a man ejaculates each time he has sex, it is like taking oil from a lamp that is already nearly burned out. Sun Ssu-mo sums up by saying that "if a man wastes his semen, he will soon die. For men, this is the most significant thing to remember about sex."

By the same token, and in agreement with the Plain Girl, Dr. Sun counsels against total abstinence. The man who has no sexual intercourse with women is prone to restlessness and longs for female companionship. Suppressing the natural urge to expel semen on occasion not only requires great effort but in fact makes it easier to lose semen. This can occur during sleep through nocturnal emissions, or so-called wet dreams. A single nocturnal ejaculation is equivalent to one hundred emissions during normal intercourse. Sun Ssu-mo suggests regulating ejaculation according to one's age, in the following manner:

1. By thirty a man begins to lose vitality and should stop wasting semen in a reckless manner. Masturbation should be forsaken and the man should become acquainted with the Tao of yin and yang.

2. By forty a man has reached a pivotal point in his life. To prevent quickly going downhill straight into the grave, which undisciplined sex causes at this stage in life, ejaculation control should become a habit.

3. By fifty a man's ejaculation should be reduced to no more than once every twenty days.

4. At sixty most men should totally curtail ejaculation (but not intercourse). A man who is very healthy and has a strong libido, however, can continue ejaculating about once a month or, even better, once in every one hundred coitions.

5. This program can continue right on through the seventies.

Ejaculation control is important for strong, healthy males as well as for those who are elderly or not so strong. Beginning such a program early in life helps avoid the worst ravages of old age, including the loss of vital energy (for more details see *Taoist Secrets of Love* by Mantak Chia and *The Multi-Orgasmic Man* by Mantak Chia and Douglas Abram).

Total celibacy for most men is equally as harmful as excessive emission. It creates a strong desire for sex, which causes an imbalance of essence, energy, and spirit. Furthermore, it ultimately causes even more loss of sexual essence and energy through the uncontrollable, intense emissions during "wet dreams." For those who wish to determine their own emission schedule, the methods of semen retention introduced in the next sections must be mastered. Then follow the guidelines given above using a trial-and-error assessment of your own vitality. A man should feel as light and refreshed after ejaculating as a woman feels after orgasm. He should not be exhausted, drained, and uninterested in more sex. An ejaculation of this sort may be experienced only when the semen supply is what the Chinese term "full" and "flourishing." If an emission leaves a man tired and depressed, he should add to the interval between ejaculations.

A man may also help reduce the loss of essence and energy because of semen emission by training himself to "come lightly" on those occasions when he chooses to ejaculate. Instead of rushing headlong to a fury just before ejaculation, advance to the edge slowly and softly and enjoy the wonderful sensation of release. Following that, intentionally "squeeze off" the urogenital canal with a heavy contraction of the anus and penis before the ejaculation is complete. This will preserve 20 to 30 percent of the semen while still giving the desired ejaculation. Right after ejaculation, rhythmically tighten the urogenital diaphragm for one or two minutes by locking the anal sphincter. This tightens the floor of the pelvis, which gets loose and slack after ejaculation. This practice helps avoid postcoital loss of Chi through the perineum, anus, and urogenital canal. This practice is very helpful for women, too, because it precludes loss of Chi through the vagina and boosts sexual energy up the spinal channels to the brain.

Many men are skeptical about this disciplined, unconventional approach to sexual relations. They need to be completely convinced by personal experience that it is a necessity. Here are a few guidelines and easy experiments any man may try to prove the truth of Tao in sex.

1. Try having vigorous intercourse shortly before taking part in an athletic event or stage performance. Do it on one occasion with ejaculation and on another without and compare the resulting performances. The difference is amazing.

2. Or have intercourse late at night, on one occasion with and on another without ejaculation. Compare the amount of sleep you need after each occasion and how you feel when you get up the next morning.

3. An even more striking test is the difference in energy felt during the day after having intercourse upon waking up in the morning. Make sure to try it both with and without ejaculation. There are numerous factors that can be checked; for example, mood, energy level, and physical condition.

4. You will definitely notice a huge difference in how you feel after having sex with or without ejaculation on an extremely cold day in the middle of winter. You will have a clear understanding of why Peng-Tze, who transcribed the *Plain Girl* text, says, "One ejaculation in winter is one hundred times more harmful than one in the spring."

5. Those who significantly reduce their ejaculation frequencies in the winter without reducing sexual intercourse are far less likely to suffer from colds, influenza, chills, the winter "blues," and other symptoms that often accompany cold weather.

6. Furthermore, if you're feeling "down and out" already, an ejaculation will only pull you deeper into depression. Having a lovemaking session without emitting semen is a terrific way to "pull yourself up" again.

7. The same principle is true in regard to physical condition. When a man is sick, losing semen only aggravates his condition by robbing him of his biggest source of resistance at the

very time he needs it most. On the other hand, disciplined intercourse mitigates a lot of chronic illnesses, especially those affected by hormone levels. Some prominent and respected celebrities have stated in interviews that they arrived at these conclusions in exactly the same way—by trial and error. You can do the same thing.

Each man must determine his own ideal rate of semen emission. It is important to know whether it is appropriate to ejaculate or not in a given situation. The calendar can help you decide whether it is suitable. One thing is quite clear, however. If a man is drunk or filled with food or sick, it is best to forgo that short-lived spasm of enjoyment and maintain one's energy. The Taoist text *Essentials for Nurturing Life* warns us that ejaculation is strictly forbidden for a man who is drunk or gorged with food. Discharges at times like this injure a man a hundred times more than under normal conditions and, indeed, may bring about dizziness and ugly genital sores.

Mastering the Techniques of Controlled Contact

All Taoist health regimens, including ejaculation control, involve the Three Treasures of essence (body), energy (breath), and spirit (mind). They are used in conjunction in an effort toward a single goal. The *Yellow Emperor's Classic* says that "spirit directs energy, energy commands essence," which means that the true Taoist man uses his mind to control his breath, breath to control blood, and blood to control semen. This is because "when blood halts, semen must halt as well." Ejaculation is always preceded by a quick speeding up of the heart. This tells us the importance of keeping the pulse normal during intercourse. Because breathing controls heartbeat, the primary exercise for developing ejaculation mastery is deep, rhythmic, abdominal breathing done in the same way as during breathing exercises (see Chapter 9).

When you lose track of your breathing, your heart rate increases, which puts you ever closer to the edge of ejaculation. It takes a few years of practice to master total voluntary control over body, breath, and mind while having sex. There are, however, some clever tricks invented by ancient practitioners to help fellow

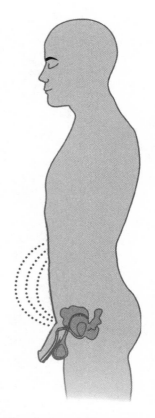

ABDOMINAL BREATHING

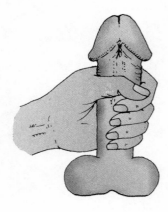

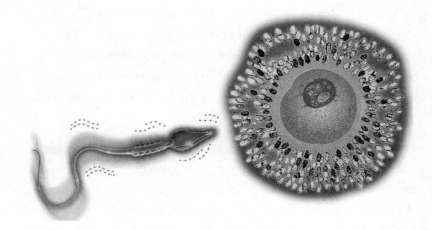

PENIS MASSAGE WITH SEMEN AND EGG

Taoists to regain control over their semen when they feel they are on the verge of ejaculating. The most important are breath retention and "locking up" the entire sacral area with tight contractions of the urogenital diaphragm. (The Taoist physician Lee Tung-hsuan talks about this in *Mysterious Master of the Cave*.) The exercise practices of the sexual organs will help stimulate the reflexology points of the sexual glands and organs, which will strengthen them. When feeling on the verge of ejaculation, a man should always hold back, at least until the woman has reached orgasm. He should remove the jade stem (penis) a little and put it between the lute strings (frenulum—just below the clitoris) and wheat buds (labia minora). He should shut his eyes, think about his mind, push his tongue against the roof of his mouth, arch his back, and stretch out his neck. Then he opens his nostrils wide, closes his mouth, and takes in a very deep breath. Doing this soon enough will postpone ejaculation.

Ejaculatory Control Practice

These are the steps to follow in controlling ejaculation. You should learn and practice controlling ejaculation alone, then apply it to dual cultivation (with your partner).

1. Once the feeling for reaching orgasm becomes strong, flex the PC muscle, also called the Chi muscle, as tightly as possible, breathing in deeply through the mouth.

2. Visualize the semen contracting back into the body while continually squeezing the Chi muscle tighter and tighter. Perform this again, massaging yourself until you feel that ejaculation is inevitable.

3. Once you are sure you are going to climax, squeeze the Chi muscle as hard as you can while breathing in through the mouth deeply. Continue to tighten the PC muscle to keep from ejaculating.

4. Begin the exercise again. Throughout the exercise, visualize the semen starting over, then contracting back into the brain until the urge subsides. Continue to squeeze the Chi muscle tighter until the urge to ejaculate has vanished. Do this ejaculatory control exercise ten times, making sure not to ejaculate during the exercise.

5. If you do ejaculate, you need to develop the Chi muscle much more. Pages 126–127 have exercises for strengthening the PC muscle.

6. Once the ejaculatory control exercise has taken its toll on you after ten to twenty sets, perform this exercise as many times as it takes to completely exhaust the Chi muscle. Achieve an erection and flex the Chi muscle a few times while you massage the penis to make sure it is quite hard.

7. Once you have a firm erection, squeeze lightly around the penis's shaft, right underneath the head. Now flex the Chi muscle as deeply as you can until it flutters, then unflex. When you flex the Chi muscle you should be able to feel the penis throb.

8. Continue to do this over and over again until the erection becomes soft. Achieve another erection, and follow the directions from steps 6-8 over and over again.

You should perform these exercises every day or at least four times a week. You will find that performing them every day makes you feel more fit and potent. Chi muscle exercises are the most important exercises you can do for penile fitness and strength development. Having a strong Chi muscle will enable you to

EJACULATORY CONTROL

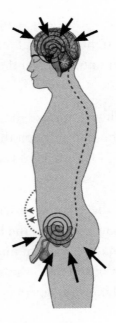
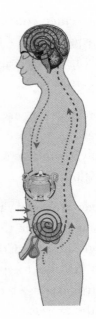

experience a whole new level of ecstasy when making love with your partner. Imagine having the ability to actually make your erections hard and keep from ejaculating by simply flexing your Chi muscle so tightly that it closes off the ejaculatory canal. If you are ready to wake up every morning with hard erections and increase your ability to perform as long as you want in lovemaking, then work on your Chi muscle. And drawing the sexual energy through the Microcosmic Orbit movement to the brain increases sexual hormones to revitalize the brain.

Breathing Exercise

As mentioned earlier, ejaculatory control is related to controlling the heart rate, which is in turn controlled by breathing. Practice this breathing exercise often, and use it to aid in ejaculation control.

1. Clear your mind of everything, including worries, problems, work, school, relationship troubles, everything.

2. Inhale through your nose as deeply as you possibly can. When you feel that you've reached your lungs' maximum capacity, keep trying until you cannot breathe in any more.

3. Hold the breath for a few seconds, and exhale through your mouth slowly, taking three to four seconds to exhale fully.

4. Repeat this for as long as you feel able; do this throughout the whole day, while driving, working, playing, and so on. You will feel much more alert. Try to do this for at least twenty minutes a day.

Buttocks Exercise

When you make love with your partner, 90 percent of your thrusting power and ability comes from your buttocks. This simple and easy exercise will strengthen, tone, and shape your gluteals for maximum sexual ability and performance, not to mention a better-looking backside. You can do this exercise anywhere.

1. Stand up with your feet facing forward about shoulder length apart.

2. In this upright position, flex and tense your buttocks as tightly as you can. Hold for ten seconds and release. Do this again five times to warm up. By now your buttocks should feel a slight burn, and that is good.

3. Now lie down on your back on the floor. With your hands to your side, flex your buttocks as tightly as you can and hold it for thirty seconds. Once you have released, flex and relax your buttocks rapidly, without stopping until you feel total fatigue and cannot flex anymore.

4. You should feel a total burn all over your buttocks; this is what you are trying to accomplish. Rest for thirty seconds, then repeat this five more times.

5. By now your buttocks should feel totally exhausted, but the workout isn't over yet. Now flex as hard as you can and hold it. Watch the clock or your wristwatch and hold this for one minute, no matter how difficult it gets! This is where your shaping and strength are going to come from, this precise exercise. After the one minute is up, without resting, repeatedly flex and unflex your buttocks for one minute. If you can,

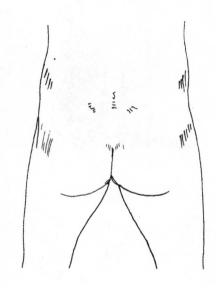

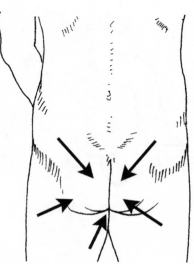

BUTTOCK SQUEEZING

WARMING THE STOVE

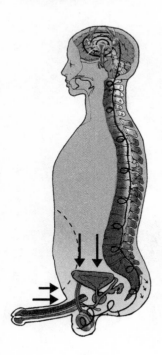

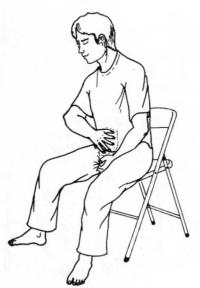

repeat this process again, holding for one minute and flexing for one minute. You should do four sets of these. Do what you can in the beginning, and continually push beyond what you think you can do until you really can't do anymore. Within a month, you should be able to do three or four times as much as you can in the beginning.

Warming the Stove (for Men)

This method of increasing sexual potency is sometimes called the Deer exercise, alluding to the abundance of sexual energy of the deer.

1. To perform this exercise, stand in a wide stance or sit on the edge of a chair.

2. Rub the palms together until warm.

3. With one hand, cup the scrotum; with the other hand, rub the lower abdomen, first clockwise and then in a counter-clockwise direction.

4. This should be done one hundred to three hundred times for optimum benefit. When the Chi moves, some people will belch or move gas.

MENSTRUAL CYCLE MANAGEMENT

Women lose their vital essence through menstruation (whereas men lose it through ejaculation). The exercises in this section enable a woman to shorten the length of her bleeding time, reduce cramping, etc. She is reabsorbing the ovarian Chi in these exercises, thus enhancing the life force in her body, rather than losing it through menstruation.

Ovary Massage

The ovarian massage is the first way to transform the menstrual cycle into life force. This is a great way to bring the female sexual energy into the whole body. It also regulates the menstrual cycle and balances hormones.

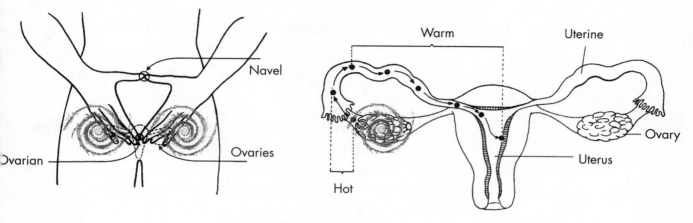

OVARY MASSAGE

1. Stand or sit upright and warm up with a few minutes of deep abdominal breathing. Massage the hands together vigorously until warm.

2. Place the hands separately over the ovaries in the lower abdomen and begin massaging the area over the ovaries in a circular clockwise motion about thirty-six times.

3. Reverse the direction. The Chi (ovarian energy) as it leaves the ovary is hot, and will become warm as it travels through the fallopian tubes to the uterus. Next, simply leave the hands resting on the ovaries, feeling the warmth penetrate the skin, energizing the entire area.

4. End with a few Chi muscle contractions (see Chapter 9) and at least one minute of deep breathing. Do this exercise two or three times daily, in order to stimulate circulation and bring healing energy into these areas.

Breast Massage

When the ovarian energy is moved up into the breasts it transforms the body. The menstrual cycle is reduced or stopped—thus successfully transforming the blood into life force or Chi.

1. Sit comfortably with the back straight or stand with feet about shoulder width apart.

2. Rub palms together until warm; place the center of the palms or the fingertips firmly over the nipples and slowly massage in circles, thirty-six times in each direction.

3. As you massage, focus your attention on the heart area, feeling the warmth of the hands radiating into the heart.

This exercise is extremely beneficial for frigidity or low libido, because it stimulates the entire endocrine system. The breast massage should be performed daily as a way to balance the hormones and menstrual cycle. It is a good exercise to prevent cysts, tumors, and breast cancer.

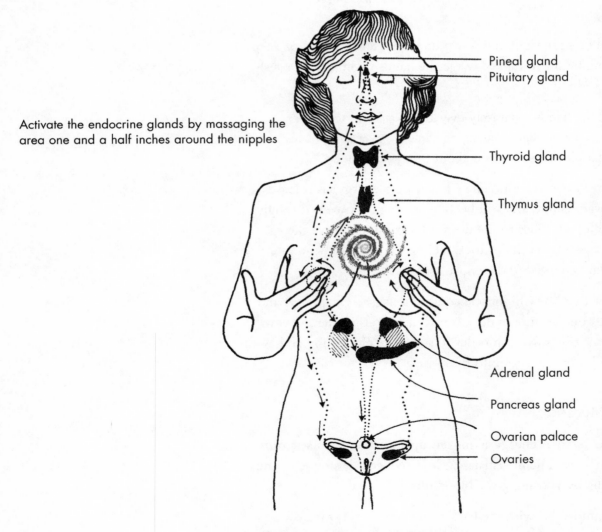

Activate the endocrine glands by massaging the area one and a half inches around the nipples

Pineal gland
Pituitary gland

Thyroid gland

Thymus gland

Adrenal gland

Pancreas gland

Ovarian palace

Ovaries

**BREAST MASSAGE—TRANSFORMING
BLOOD INTO CHI**

EGG EXERCISES AND VAGINAL WEIGHT LIFTING

The use of a stone egg to strengthen the vagina is a practice that evolved in ancient China. As time went on, the secret of this practice remained in the Royal Palace and was taught only to the queen and concubines. Many who mastered the technique experienced very good health, remaining young and bountiful, with sexual organs in old age as tight and resilient as those of a young, unmarried woman. Some believe that the queen and concubines practiced the technique in order to please the king while making love. Originally, however, the Egg exercise and Vaginal Weight Lifting were implemented for improving health, both physically and spiritually, since these exercises provide more power to the Chi muscle to lift the sexual energy inward and upward, where it can be transformed into higher spiritual energy.

The egg is a marvelous way to strengthen and control the Chi muscle. It is easier to practice control of this muscle with an egg in the vagina, since, as the egg moves, you can feel more distinctly the direction in which the Chi muscle moves. Controlling this voluntary muscle means control of the many involuntary muscles in this area as well. Also, as you master the use of this muscle of the vagina and perineum, you simultaneously tone up the lower abdomen. This will in turn increase the flow of sexual hormones, and greatly improve your performance of Ovarian Breathing, the Orgasmic Upward Draw, and the Organs' Orgasm (for more details, see *Healing Love through the Tao* by Mantak Chia).

Vaginal Weight Lifting is a very powerful practice to strengthen, in addition to the Chi muscle, the urogenital and pelvic diaphragms. The strength of these two diaphragms is very important, since they serve as floors to the sexual organs and all vital organs. When the Chi muscle and diaphragms become loose, Chi pressure will leak out from the organs as they stack up on each other, dropping all their weight to rest upon the perineum. When strengthened, the muscle and the diaphragms function as before, preventing leakage of life force and sexual energies. (Note: Eggs can be purchased from the Universal Tao, their local instructors, or a gem shop. Do not use a real egg!)

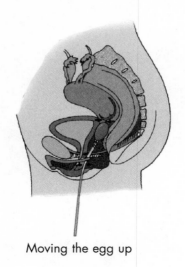

Moving the egg up

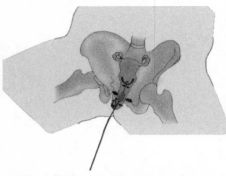

Using both sections to move the egg sideways

EGG EXERCISE WITH ONE EGG

Egg Exercise

1. **Insert the egg:** When you feel you are ready, insert the egg into the vagina, large end first.

2. **Horse Stance alignment:** Align your body in the Horse Stance (standing with feet slightly wider than hip width apart, knees slightly bent).

3. **Contract the bottom section of the vagina:** Isolate and contract the muscle groups responsible for closing the external vaginal orifice tightly. This will help to keep the egg in the vaginal canal.

4. **Contract the top section:** Inhale and contract the vaginal canal muscles immediately in front of the cervix so that you are now contracting two sections at the same time. Keep both points closed. There is no need to use hard muscle contractions. The strength required depends a great deal on the control of these muscles, which you have gained by practicing the vaginal weight-lifting exercises.

5. **Squeeze the middle section:** Slightly squeeze the egg from the middle of the vaginal canal until you feel that you have a good grip on it. Inhale and squeeze again, gradually increasing the squeeze, and then inhale more and squeeze harder. Once you feel you have a really firm grip on the egg, slowly move it up and down. Start with a slow motion, gradually increasing to a fast motion. When you are out of breath, exhale and rest. The resting period is very important. It is at this time that you will feel Chi build up in this area. Try to master each movement before continuing to the next. Use the top section to move the egg horizontally: Next, move the egg left and right still using the top section. Practice until you master this action.

6. **Use the bottom section to move the egg horizontally:** Next move the egg left and right from the bottom. Using the mind together with some muscle movement is important, since you cannot move the egg with hard muscle contractions alone. There are many involuntary muscles within the vaginal canal, which the mind and Chi muscle help to move.

7. **Use both sections to move the egg horizontally:** Now move the egg left and right as you wish, holding it by the top and bottom muscles. Master this before continuing to the next step.

8. **Use both sections to tilt the egg:** Next tilt the egg forward and back (toward the front of the body and then the back of the body), using the top and the bottom sections of the vagina. Master this action.

9. **Combine all movements:** Combine all these movements, moving the egg left and right, tilting it forward and backward, moving it up to touch the cervix and then down to the external vaginal orifice. Rest. All during the Egg Exercise, the contraction of the vaginal canal in the area in front of the cervix activating the pineal gland and the external orifice is to remain constant until you have finished moving the egg. This particular egg exercise should be practiced two to three times per week. You may perform this very same exercise daily without actually inserting the egg by following the same sequence using the contractile strength of the vaginal muscles to suck in an imaginary egg and move it up, down, left, and right.

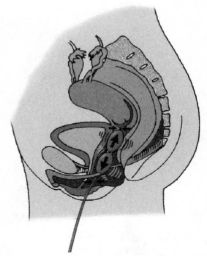

Squeezing two eggs apart

Jade eggs are ideal for these exercises and come in two sizes, small and big. The small one is less than an inch wide and one-and-a-half inches long; the bigger is wider than an inch and slightly longer than the small egg. To enhance your development, you should begin by using a small egg. As you progress, the larger egg may be used to mark the progress in your "sucking" abilities. You may wish to further develop your skill by using two eggs. Eventually the practice of egg sucking will become so mastered that you will be able to suck the egg into the vagina from the outside with a vacuumlike motion. Such a powerful sucking ability enhances experiences in your life such as childbearing or lovemaking. Imagine the intense pleasure of your lover as he discovers your "third hand" while you demonstrate to him your power and skill.

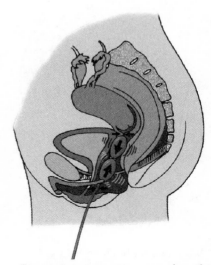

Squeezing two eggs toward each other

EGG EXERCISE WITH TWO EGGS

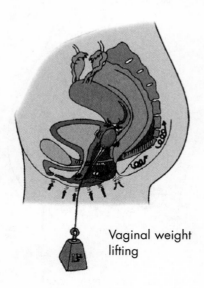

Vaginal weight lifting

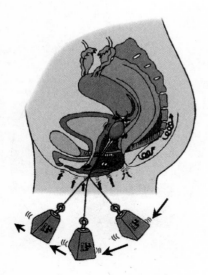

Vaginal weight lifting and swing

CHI VAGINAL WEIGHT LIFTING

Vaginal Weight Lifting

For these exercises you will need to use a stone egg with a small opening at each end through which a string can be passed. You should use minimal weights to start and slowly increase. To prepare for insertion of the egg, massage your breasts in the manner prescribed earlier in this chapter, and massage the external genitals.

1. **Tie the string to the weight:** After the string has been passed through the egg and secured with a knot at the egg's large end, tie the weight (a fishing weight, under a pound, is good to start) to the string. If the weight has no attaching point, it can also be placed inside a bag or container attached to the string. A weight holder can also be used, first without any weight, and then with the gradual addition of a holding clamp and the weight. Either place a chair in front of you and rest the weight on it, or place the weight on the floor and squat down to facilitate the egg's insertion (remember to support the weight with your fingers).

2. **Insert the egg:** Kneel down near where the weight is resting and insert the egg into the vagina, large end first (use a lubricant if necessary but not too much as you will not be able to grip the egg). Close the vagina, contracting the muscles around the egg to hold it. Slowly rise to stand with your feet a hip width apart.

3. **Swing the weight:** Swinging the weight gives the practitioner control over the amount of pressure on the groin, which is why lighter weights are recommended initially. The Chi from the fascial connection between the perineum and the kidneys is used to pull the weight. In the beginning, swing the weights front to back gently as you determine the amount of pressure that is comfortable for you.

   Inhale as you contract the anus and perineum. Swing the attached weight from thirty-six to forty-nine times. Synchronize your breathing with each swing. Inhale as the weight swings backward, between the legs, and exhale as it swings forward, away from the legs. Pull up against the weight internally with each forward swing, and draw the energy up to the coccyx, the sacrum, and eventually all the way through the crown to the pineal gland. Each completed swing back and forth should approximate one second.

After a week, try to swing the weight for sixty counts. More pressure results from the counterforce exerted by the Chi muscle when heavier weights are swung, but it is wiser to increase this pressure by using lighter weights and adding more power to each swing. Do this by rocking the pelvis, putting more energy into the movement. The lighter weights should be used to their maximum potential, thereby strengthening the Chi muscle and producing more hormones.

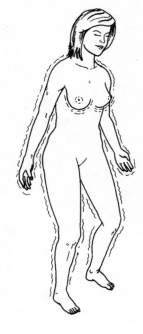

PHYSICAL SEXERCISES

The physical sexercises are different from a normal workout. Most of these would not be appropriate at your local fitness or workout club. These exercises focus specifically on the sexual organs and pelvis. Over time, just as with any other workout, the strength in this area will dramatically increase. This benefits the whole body, including the mind and the emotions, as sexual health is uplifting to the totality of the individual.

Shaking the Testicles and the Breasts

Shaking the body is a fantastic way to open the meridians. Shaking different parts of the body brings circulation and release of tension. This exercise should be performed naked or with loose clothing.

1. The feet should be a bit wider than shoulder width apart.

2. Start bouncing gently up and down as if there were a large Chi ball in the center of your belly, and when you bounce, it bounces. Feel all the joints shake loose, the wrists, elbows, shoulders, hips, and spine.

3. For men, this should cause the penis and the testicles to bounce up and down, and they should feel loose.

4. For women, the hopping should cause the breasts to bounce. Feel the sexual organs loose and relaxed.

Continue for at least two minutes at first and eventually longer

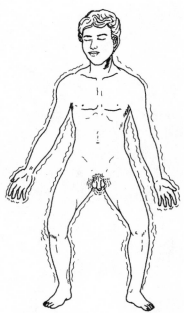

SHAKING THE TESTICLES AND BREASTS

as your stamina increases. For men, this exercise strongly stimulates the testicles, penis, and prostate. For women, it stimulates the ovaries and enhances blood circulation to the sexual center.

Spiraling Hip and Tailbone (for Men and Women)

The sacrum can and does move separately from the hips. This may take a while to feel and do. Start by sitting and with intention hold the hips steady while turning the sacrum first left and then right. Imagine the sacrum spiraling as if you had a tail.

1. This exercise is performed in a wide stance, with the hands on the hips or extended in front of the body. Allow the breath to be full and deep, without any specific relation to the movement. Spiral the tailbone, or coccyx, and sacrum separately from the hips, first in a clockwise direction, extending the hips forward and backward as far as possible.

2. Reverse the direction. Let the movement be relaxed and free, feeling the joints of the hips loosen and stretch.

This exercise relaxes and strengthens the tailbone, hips, and lower back, allowing the sacrum more range of motion and increasing circulation in the sexual center. Spiraling the tailbone

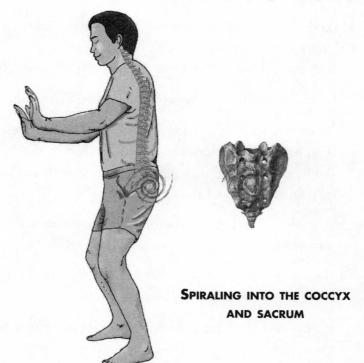

SPIRALING INTO THE COCCYX AND SACRUM

stimulates and stretches the nerve fibers in the sacral region, activating the hormones of the testicles, ovaries, prostate, and uterus. As the Taoists say, the genitals get stuck together in the sacrum. By spiraling the hips you will open this area up and unlock the genitals.

Secret Taoist Method of Urination (for Men and Women)

An exercise that greatly strengthens the PC muscle is the Urination Exercise. The practice of this exercise is also designed to strengthen the kidneys, the organs and tendons which, according to Chinese medicine, regulate sexual function. Therefore, in order to increase one's sexual potential, it is very important to strengthen the kidneys. This exercise helps cure premature ejaculation and impotence when practiced over a period of time and helps to prevent incontinence in women. It is a simple exercise that consists of stopping the flow of urine by contraction of the PC muscle while urinating.

1. When you have a full bladder, begin by urinating normally, then contract the Chi muscle, stopping the flow of urine.

2. Now exhale, pressing the lower abdomen, and feel pressure on the bladder. Then start to urinate and again contract the Chi muscle.

3. Hold for about three seconds and resume urination. While doing this exercise, raise up and lower your heels three to five times per urination.

4. Doing this exercise a few times a day greatly strengthens the urogenital diaphragm, all the body tendons, and sexual energy.

Sun Practice (for Men and Women)

Being naked in the sun is a wonderful way to reenergize the whole body. According to the Taoist masters, our bodies can in fact absorb energy from nature. That is why we feel so much more alive at the beach, in the woods, or near a lake. For example, just think about where you usually want to go on a vacation. It is probably somewhere out in or near nature, because of the abundance of energy.

A powerful Taoist exercise is to absorb the rays of the sun into the genitals. Find a place in your backyard, or even in your house where the sun can enter through an open window, and sit or stand comfortably, allowing the rays of the sun to shine on the genitals. Feel the warmth energize and relax the pelvic area. Breathe deeply into the lower abdomen. The morning or late-afternoon sun is preferable to the midday sun (11:00 A.M. to 1:00 P.M.), which is too strong. The practice takes only five to ten minutes or not too much longer. Burning the parts of your body where the sun normally doesn't shine is not much fun, so be careful.

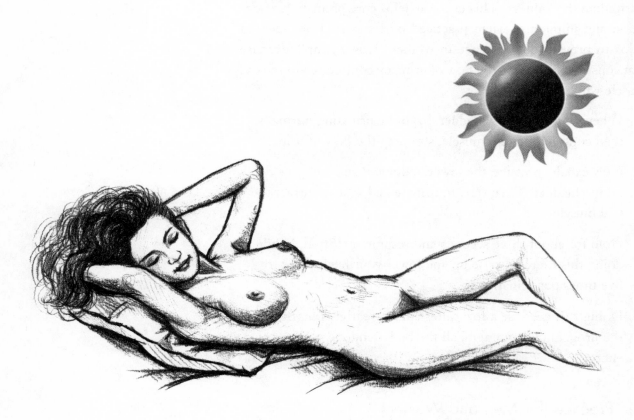

SUN PRACTICE

Sexual Reflexology and Physical Characteristics

The study of sexual reflexology and physical characteristics will help you determine the sexual potential and physical compatibility of another person. Sexual reflexology enables you to evaluate a person's internal energy levels, as well as the size and shape of the person's sexual organs, by combining and observing the external characteristics, beginning with physical appearances of the face and continuing to other bodily features, such as the hair, neck, fingers and hands, and color and structure of the body. The following section will help reveal the strengths and weaknesses of a person as well as compatibility between couples.

All external features of the body are helpful in determining the sexual compatibility of a partner's and one's own internal energy.

Yet it is important to remember that these are only guidelines and many factors need to be taken into consideration before one can really understand another person's capabilities. With practice, one can become skilled at recognizing the sexual inclinations and capacities of others; the recommendations in this book are merely suggestions to help one in the beginning.

TAOIST SEXUAL TERMS

The Taoists use poetic phrases to indicate the beauty and sacred aspect of the body and sexual organs. The terms used here demonstrate the reverence for the sexual organs and the physical body itself. In the West, sexuality is often referred to derogatorily and the sexual organs treated as something dirty and degrading. This attitude creates an array of emotional problems revolving around our sexual nature and relationships in general. If we start to view our sexual energy and sexual organs as sacred, as a source of vital energy, we experience great satisfaction with others and ourselves.

Here is a list of Taoist terms for our sexuality:

Vagina	*Hidden palace*
	Valley of solitude
	Celestial palace
	Path of yin
	Cinnabar cave
	Vermilion cave
Breasts	*Bells of love*
Penis	*Jade stalk*
	Yang peak
	Ambassador
Testicles	*Dragon pearls*
Intercourse	*Clouds and rain*
Clitoris	*Precious pearl*
	Yin bean
	Jade terrace
Cunnilingus	*Sipping the vast spring*
Fellatio	*Blowing the flute*
Orgasm	*High tide*

FACIAL FEATURES

Lips

For some men, a woman's lips may be one of her most attractive physical features. It is said that when a woman wins her lover's affection with her eyes, this love is an intellectual affair. But when she wins her love's affection with her lips, it is a passionate affair. Thus the eyes indicate a more intellectual orientation, while the lips indicate a more emotional orientation. In addition, although it can be said that a man or a woman may use his or her eyes to seduce a partner, it is the lips that will determine the nature of the relationship.

The shape of the lips reveals the health of the body. Some lips are full, not necessarily large or small. They have a curved, symmetric outline, without drooping or slackness. This reveals strong, healthy organs and sexual energy. When the upper lip arches upward and the lower lip folds downward, creating a slight hollow under the lower lip, this indicates harmony between the ring muscles and the internal organs.

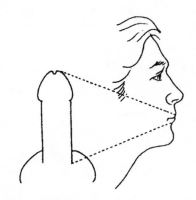

Thin small lips indicate a short penis

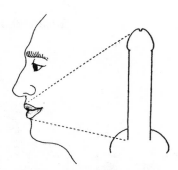

Wide and thick lips indicate a long penis

**RELATIONSHIP OF LIPS
AND PENIS SIZE**

- It is believed that the upper lip relates to the nature of giving love, while the lower lip relates to the nature of receiving love. A person with a plusher, more protruding upper lip is usually more giving or aggressive in giving affection, while a person with a fatter, plusher, and more protruding lower lip will be more likely to enjoy receiving affection than giving it.

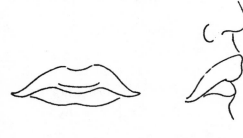

The upper lip relates to the nature of giving love; a protruding upper lip denotes a more giving personality

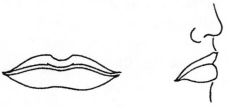

The lower lip relates more to the nature of receiving love; a lower lip that is larger than the upper lip indicates the person will be more likely to enjoy receiving affection than giving it

SIZE AND SHAPE OF LIPS

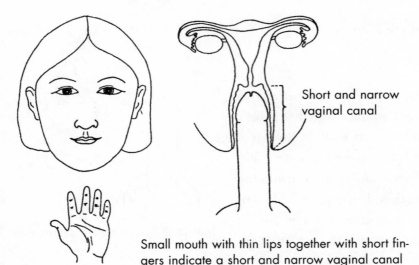

Short and narrow vaginal canal

Small mouth with thin lips together with short fingers indicate a short and narrow vaginal canal

SHORT VAGINAL CANAL

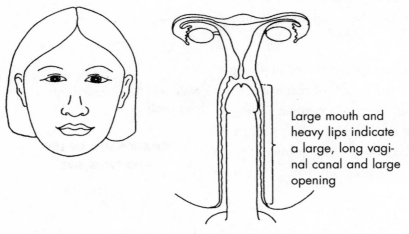

Large mouth and heavy lips indicate a large, long vaginal canal and large opening

LONG VAGINAL CANAL

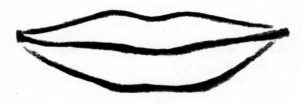

LARGE MOUTH

- Those persons whose lower lip is especially sensitive to touch will usually fall in love and enjoy sex before engaging in an intellectual relationship with their lover.

- To be effective in the stimulation of one's partner, the lips must be moist. A sign of sexual arousal in both men and women is when either partner licks his or her lips, indicating that the person is ready for a sexual encounter. In the classics this was called "preparing the field to be plowed."

- The mouth and genitals are considered opposite poles of the body, and as such, one is regarded as the reflection of the other. Thus, when a person talks incessantly, this indicates that the person is sexually frustrated and the energy is channeled through conversation rather than sexual expression.

- If the person has a large mouth, it indicates that the person has a tendency to scream aloud during orgasm and has a large capacity for sex.

Erotic kissing, involving the lips and tongue, is a part of love play. When couples kiss with their tongues in what is commonly referred to as a soul kiss or French kissing, the tongue directly reflects and connects their hearts, while their lips give and receive affection between each other. Also, the Governor and Functional channels of each partner both connect at the lips and tongue, making a complete circuit of energy flow when the couple kisses.

FRENCH KISSING

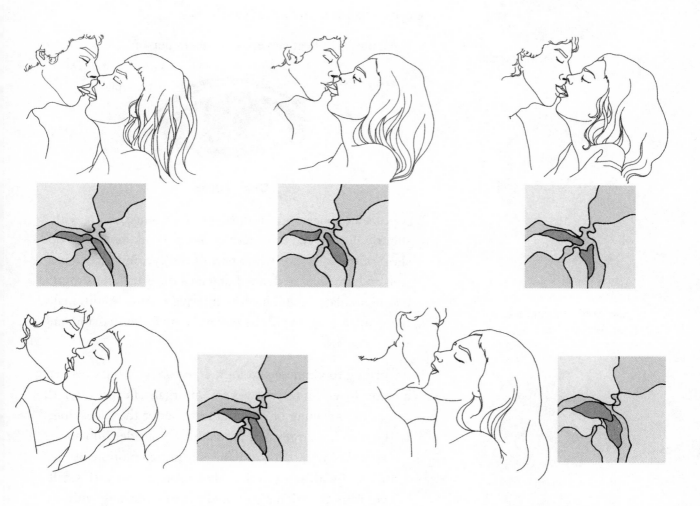

Eyes

There is a strong connection between the eyes and the sexual center. The ring muscles in the eyes correlate with the ring muscles in the urogenital diaphragm. A wink between a couple, for example, affects the ring muscles around the sexual organs; hence the

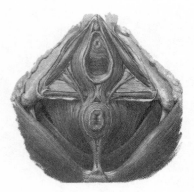

External anal sphincter muscles of female

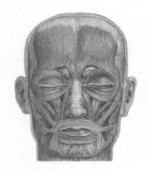

The sphincter muscles in the face connect to the anal sphincter and the genital sphincter muscle

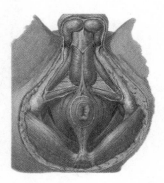

External anal sphincter muscle of male

RING MUSCLE OF THE EYES AND SEXUAL ORGANS

erotic significance of the wink in folklore. Winking gently activates the sexual energy.

In Chinese medicine, the eyes are considered the windows to a person's soul and physically are connected to the liver. They can be used for diagnosis of internal disorders but are also the vehicles through which love and sexual potential can be detected. Following are some of the sexual behavior signals emanating from the eyes, according to Chinese analyses.

1. Dark pupils indicate a very passionate person.

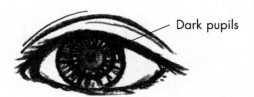

Dark pupils

DARK PUPILS

2. A peaceful appearance in the eyes of a woman, along with a slightly flushed red tint (perhaps faintly pink, but not bloodshot) of the sclera, or white part of the eye, indicates a passionate individual with an abundance of sexual energy, good blood circulation, and healthy internal organs. Additionally, the woman's vagina will be warm owing to her passion and sexual desires.

3. According to Chinese sexology, a person with big eyes makes a better lover. Since the eyes are an organ of expression, they can emote a feeling or communicate better than speaking.
   a. If a man has large eyes, the Chinese consider him an expert in love affairs, in that he is more emotionally involved with sex. On the other hand, a man with small eyes is more rational and intellectual in dealing with sex and women.
   b. A woman with big eyes is usually more outgoing and open-minded. This may make her more receptive to male advances. A Chinese proverb says, "A lady with big eyes cannot be a poor sex partner." Since the eyes are the windows of the soul, big eyes indicate a love of life, action, and passion.

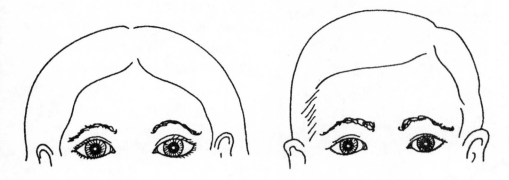

Large eyes indicate superior lovers

SIZE OF EYES

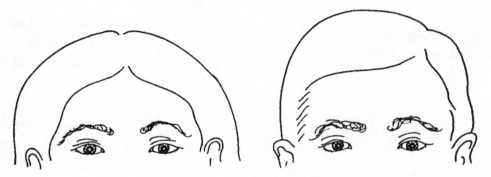

Small eyes indicate a rational mind

Eyebrows

The eyebrows, according to Chinese Taoist sexuality, express one's inner feelings of love, inner personality, and inner sexuality. The eyebrows are full of expression, especially in women, usually revealing their emotional state.

Observe the nature of the eyebrows in different situations: shocked, scared, surprised, and so on. Notice how they show the state of the emotion being expressed; for example, contracted eyebrows indicate sorrow or worry. "Flying and dancing" eyebrows indicate joy and excitement. Small and narrow eyebrows indicate sorrow and sadness. In the Orient, the expression "making eyes and eyebrows at someone" is used, as opposed to "making eyes at someone," the Western expression. Observe pictures portraying characters from the Chinese or Japanese theater (for example, Kabuki theater) and you will see elaborate makeup, especially emphasizing the eyes and eyebrows. Modern women also use makeup on their eyes and eyebrows, and many pull hairs from their eyebrows to create a clean shape. The cosmetic industry has provided women with a wide range of eye enhancer products: eyeliner, eye shadow, eyebrow pencils, eyelash curlers, and so on. Every imaginable color and all kinds of glitter are available. This illustrates that the eyes and the eyebrows are now, as in the past, important expressions of love and attraction.

Women from East and West indicate that they observe the man's eyes as one of the prerequisites of attraction. "He has smiling eyes" or "He has bedroom eyes" or eyes "that look right through me" are not uncommon expressions in sexual attraction. If a man has eyebrows shaped like crescent moons, strongly curved rather than straight, he is more sexually oriented than intellectually oriented.

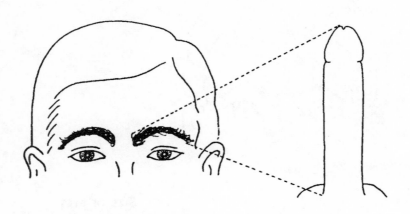

FULL LONG EYEBROWS INDICATE A STRONG, LONG PENIS

Space between the Eyebrows

The space between the eyebrows indicates levels of consciousness. It should be wide enough for another eye to fit there. As one ages, this space becomes wider, as

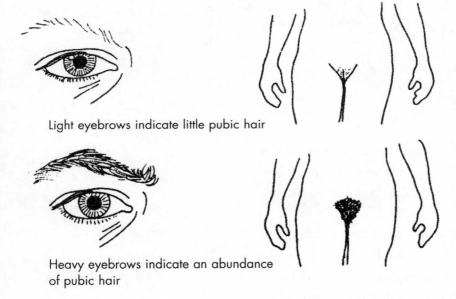

Light eyebrows indicate little pubic hair

Heavy eyebrows indicate an abundance of pubic hair

THICKNESS OF EYEBROWS

if to accommodate another eye, indicating that the person has become wiser and more tolerant. This space between the eyebrows, corresponding to the third-eye center (or pituitary gland center), also corresponds to the sexual organs. The average space between the eyebrows is one and one-half to two index-finger breadths. When this space is wider, it indicates for both men and women a strong sex drive. In women, a wide space also means a wide vagina.

Teeth

According to the ancient Taoist physicians, the aging process begins with a decline in the kidneys' and sexual organs' energy, manifesting itself in failing eyesight, decaying teeth, receding gums, inflexibility of the spine; and finally, a decline in the person's sexual potential.

The incisor teeth, or "frontal bones" in Chinese medicine, are believed to be associated with the kidneys. Since the kidneys are responsible for our sexual power or strength, it follows that the incisors are indicative of a person's sexual potential. The stomach meridian is also reflected in the upper incisors. This is significant because the stomach and spleen together are called an "ocean of food" from which all the organs and, ultimately, the body derive nourishment.

Incisors, canines, and molars should all be observed from a sexological point of view. The size of these teeth is important in judging the sexual potential of a person.

1. A person with large teeth will have a rough head of hair or body hair. This person will be passionate and sexually aggressive.

2. A woman with tiny, beautifully arranged teeth will have strong and beautifully arranged genitals and will be very sexually rewarding for her partner.

3. A man with a good set of teeth usually has strong kidneys and, consequently, strong sexual power.

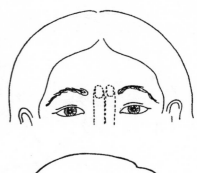

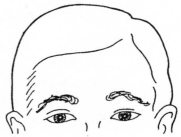

WIDE SPACE BETWEEN THE EYEBROWS INDICATES A STRONG SEX DRIVE

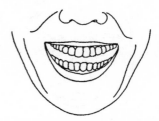

Large teeth indicate a passionate and sexually aggressive personality

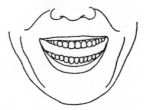

Small teeth indicate a tight vagina

SIZE OF TEETH

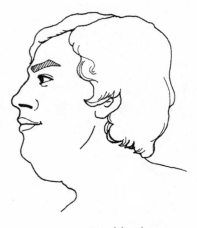

Double chin

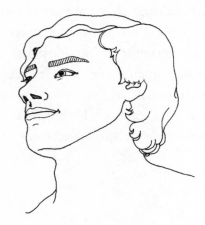

Square jaw

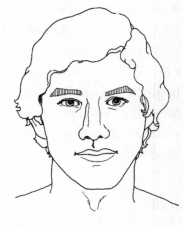

Strong jaw

JAWLINES

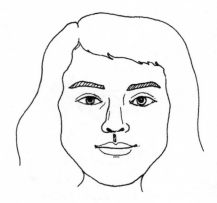

FULL CHEEKS

Jawlines

A strong jawline with good definition is indicative of a strong sexual potential for both the male and female. A person without a strong jawline (for example, with a double or triple chin), with no jawline, or with a weak jaw possesses a weaker sexual potential.

Cheeks

For the female, the cheeks are second only to the lips among facial features in importance in sexuality. The cheeks reflect the kidneys in Chinese physiognomy. When a woman's cheeks, the lower side of her face, are full, wide, and muscular (that is, firm, not loose), she has strong sexual energy.

Ears

The ears are sexually symbolic appendages, especially for a woman. By studying a woman's ears, a man will be able to determine not only the angle of her vagina but also the size and shape of it as well as aspects of her inner personality. A woman, on the other hand, can determine from a man's ears whether he is strong, robust, and healthy. She will also be able to tell if he is going to live long, be wealthy, and so on, all by observing the shape and coloration of his ears.

The ideal type of ear is one that is thick and meaty all around the circumference. The color of a healthy ear is pink and slightly transparent looking. This is a sign of good health and strong sexual potential. If a woman is shy and her ears turn red, this indicates good health. If her ears look transparent, this indicates good health, a warm personality, and good sexual potential, especially if they turn redder than her complexion at times of embarrassment or sexual excitation.

If a man's ears turn redder than his face, this indicates great sexual potential. Large, fat-lobed ears that protrude from the head also indicate good sexual potential, as well as strong kidneys and a strong constitution. He will be supplied with a great deal of kidney Chi.

A person with thin and smaller ears will be deficient in kidney energy and have weaker sexual potential.

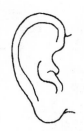

This small ear indicates deficient kidney energy and weak sexual potential

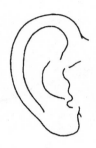

An ear that is thick and fleshy all around the rim is a sign of good health and strong sexual potency

Nose

The function of the nose, being the instrument of breath, is crucial to a healthy, vibrant body. The nostrils can activate all the sphincters (ring muscles) of the body. For example, when a healthy individual is sexually aroused, the nostrils flare open in conjunction with the breath. This activates the energy of the entire body.

1. A woman with a small nose has warmth and also the potential for many sex partners.

2. A woman with a fine, thin, bony, sharp-lined, and sharp-tipped nose is more nervous, more sensitive, loses her temper easily, and has an erratic personality.

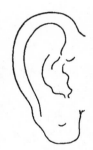

Large ears that protrude from the head, with fat lobes, indicate good sexual potential and strong kidneys

SIZE OF EARS

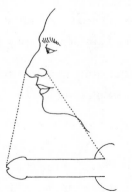

A LONG NOSE INDICATES A LONG PENIS

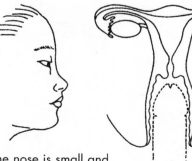

If the nose is small and flat, the vagina is wide with a short channel

A SMALL, FLAT NOSE

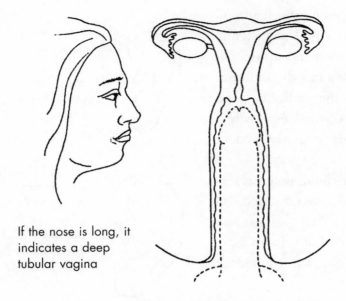

If the nose is long, it indicates a deep tubular vagina

A LONG NOSE

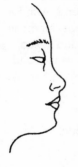

The small nose indicates a warm personality

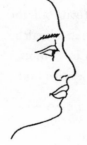

The broad, flat nose indicates a quiet, domestic, and dependent personality

SMALL AND BROAD NOSES

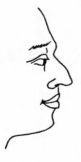

The "hawk," or hooked, nose indicates an energetic and often sexually aggressive personality

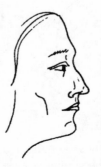

The fine, thin, bony nose indicates a sensitive, more nervous, and often erratic personality

HOOKED AND THIN NOSES

3. A woman with a broad, flat nose is more likely to be quieter, more domestic, and dependent on a man.

4. A woman with a hawk, or hook-shaped, nose is full of energy, sexually aggressive, and possibly fierce in nature.

5. A woman with a depressed root or base of the nose is very aggressive and very emotional.

Male Facial Features Summarized

1. If a man's lips are wide and thick, it is an indication of a bigger penis.

2. Thin, small lips indicate a smaller penis.

3. A thick, flat nose indicates a thick penis shaft.

4. A long nose indicates a long penis.

5. Deep eyes with thin-skinned eyelids indicate a long penis.

6. A full, long eyebrow indicates a strong, long penis.

7. If the area of the ear's conch, referred to by the Taoists as the "ditch of the ear," is deep set, it is an indication of a strong penis of good size.

8. A large, thick neck on a man indicates a very strong and thick penis.

Female Facial Features Summarized

We enter this world through the portals of the Jade Gate, and once born we seek forever to return. This eternal truth holds a message: that man's joy and vigor come from the same place as his creation.

—MING DYNASTY ANONYMOUS POEM

1. If a woman's mouth is small in width, with thin lips, she possesses a short and narrow vaginal canal. Conversely, a woman with a large, wide mouth will have a large, long, and wide vagina.

2. If a woman has thick lips, her vaginal canal is wide at the entrance and large.

3. If a woman's lips protrude, her vagina is elastic, in that it can expand to accommodate a larger penis. With ample lubrication, it is considered to be an elastic and "moving" vagina.

4. A woman with tiny, beautifully arranged teeth will also have very strong and beautifully arranged genitals. Her vagina can accommodate the penis in a perfect and tight way with no empty spaces, permitting maximum contact and friction for maximum pleasure.

5. If a woman's nose is small and flat, her vagina is wide but the canal is short.

6. If a woman's nose is long, it indicates a deep, tubular vagina.

7. A lower chin that is strong, has no extra jowls, and is muscular looking reflects a strong genital system, beautifully arranged, and a tight, muscular vagina. Remember that the proportionality and strength of the body suggest the size and shape of the genitals.

8. A woman with a slim face and muscular lower cheeks will have a vaginal wall that is thick and full of muscles.

9. Dimples indicate a short and small vagina with expanding capacity. This type of vagina can expand to accommodate a larger penis.

10. Protruding eyes indicate that the vaginal canal is short.

11. If a woman is born nearsighted, it is an indication of a short vaginal canal.

12. If the eyes are deep set, this indicates that a woman's vaginal canal is deep, or long.

13. If a woman's eyes are moist or sparkling, it means her vaginal lubrication is ample. If her eyes are dry, it means she has less vaginal lubrication; that is, the vagina is more on the dry side.

14. A full, long, moon-shaped eyebrow reveals a healthy, strong vagina with a long canal. Also, when the woman is having her period, the hairs on her eyebrows will stand up more than they normally would.

15. Sparse eyebrows on a woman indicate she has little pubic hair. If she has heavy eyebrows, she has more pubic hair.

16. A wide space between the eyebrows means a woman's vagina is wide. When sexually aroused, this space between the eyebrows can be observed to be wider than usual.

17. The shape of the "ditch" of a woman's ear (in the conch area) corresponds to the shape of her vagina and its size. A deep-set ear ditch is healthy, indicating a strong, deep vagina.

MASSAGING THE FACE

Massaging the face can be very relaxing and enticing. Opening the energy in the face activates the energy in the sexual center. Remember that the face and the sexual center are connected through the ring muscles; when one is stimulated, so is the other. Notice all the facial expressions when one is sexually excited! Stimulating the sexual center changes the facial expression, reflecting this excitement. The opposite is also true. Stimulating the face can be very erotic and stimulating to the sexual center.

Have your partner lie in your lap or between your legs so that it is easy to massage the face. No formal techniques are required, just good intention and a soft touch. Begin exploring your partner's face with a light and gentle touch. Massage around the eyes, across the forehead, over the cheeks, and around the lips. Feel the unique quality of the face. Kissing the face is another way to open the connection between the face and the sexual center. Softly kissing the cheeks, the forehead, the eyes, and the nose is very sensual and stimulating.

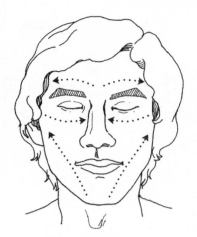

FACIAL MASSAGE

HANDS AND FINGERS

In Chinese sexology, the middle finger is considered most important in the man, while the pinkie, or little finger, is most relevant to the woman's sexuality. It is believed that a man with a long middle finger has strong sexuality, while in a woman there is a close relationship between her pinkie finger and her sexual energy. If the pinkie finger is long, she is in possession of great sexual power, her energy will be plentiful, and she will be high-spirited. The pinkie finger is associated with the heart meridian and has a strong energetic connection with the emotions and the sexual center. For men, the middle finger is associated with the pericardium, or the circulation sex meridian, and with the yang aspect of the heart.

Frequently cold hands on a woman mean a yang deficiency; conversely, warm hands indicate a great abundance of yang energy. A woman suffering from a yang energy deficiency experiences this deficiency throughout her body, possibly including her vagina. Being cold may reduce her excitability and her vaginal size. Thus a woman with cold hands may not be as passionate as one with warm hands. In having yin energy in excess, she may have vaginal lubrication, but she may have relatively less vaginal dilation.

Thin fingers are an indication of a thin penis

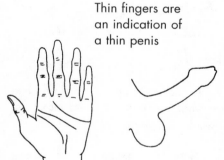

SIZE AND SHAPE OF FINGERS

Fingers of a Man

The size of a man's fingers and thumb reflects the size and shape of his penis. When discussing size and shape, it is important to remember that no one size or shape is better than another. What

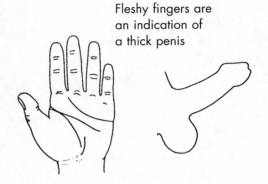

Fleshy fingers are an indication of a thick penis

SIZE AND SHAPE OF FINGERS

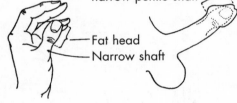

A fat thumb head indicates a fat head in the penis; a narrow shaft in the thumb indicates a narrow penile shaft

—Fat head
—Narrow shaft

A "mushroom" penis with a large head and narrow shaft is best for maximum vaginal stimulation

SIZE AND SHAPE OF THE THUMB

is important is that the size and shape be in harmony with the partner. The most important factor in sexuality is the quality of our internal energy.

1. If all of a man's fingers are fleshy, wide, or thick, it is an indication of a thick penis.

2. If all of a man's fingers are thin, it indicates a thinner penis.

3. Long fingers, especially the first finger, indicate a long penis.

4. A good-shaped thumb for a man is a fat tip with a small root, thus indicating a penis with a fat head and a thinner penile shaft. Because of its shape this is called a mushroom penis, and it is best for maximum female vaginal stimulation.

Fingers of a Woman

The size and shape of a woman's thumbs reflect the size and shape of her vagina, or vaginal canal.

1. A fat thumb head with a narrow-rooted shaft is equivalent to a tight vaginal opening with a vaginal canal that is wider on the inside. This condition is well suited for the mushroom-shaped penis.

2. A thumb that is not fat at the fingernail, or end, but more tubular in shape reflects a vagina also tubular in shape.

3. Short fingers accompany a short and narrow vaginal canal.

SIZE AND SHAPE OF WOMAN'S THUMB

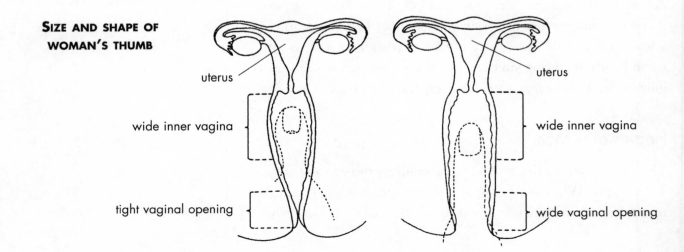

Massaging the Hands

Massaging the hands can relax the whole body. By stimulating the points on the hands, one can activate and balance sexual energy. It can be very erotic for a couple to massage each other's hands, exploring the fingers, lines, and palms. The hands are like a map revealing the unique experiences of a person. Send your loving energy through the hands. Work between the fingers, across the knuckles, and all through the center of the palms. Also, it is very stimulating to lick, suck, or kiss the hands of your partner. This elicits a very powerful current of sexual energy through the whole body.

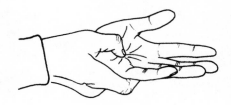

HAND MASSAGE

HAIR

According to Taoist medicine, hair on the head, eyebrow hair, and pubic hair all are related to human sexuality. For the woman, hair on her body is supported by the yin energy of the kidneys, while in the male, hair is supported by the yang energy of the kidneys. The hair on the head is directly related to the kidneys. This is because the bladder meridians traverse the top of the head. Loss of hair and premature graying are the first manifestations of a lower functioning of the kidneys and the resultant loss of kidney Chi. The kidneys, whose essence nurtures the blood, are no longer doing so efficiently, and the result is the initiation of aging. A man's baldness may also be due to a congenital weakness, bad hygiene, or inadequate diet, as well, of course, as his inherited genes or ancestral energy.

An abundance of hair is therefore a sign of strong sexuality and ample sexual energy in Taoist medicine.

A man who has abundant body hair has a strong sexual power, even if he is bald or balding on top. It seems that his body hair is formed from the excess energy of the blood and is directed, via the lung, which controls the skin, to the surface to be stored as excess body hair. Hair on the face is another sign of strong sexual power in a male. So if he has a full beard or a strong mustache, it indicates strong sexual potential.

From the *Nei Ching* (Yellow Emperor's Classic), regarding the male, we find: "If the whiskers on both cheeks are handsome and long, then the energy and blood in the upper bright yang meridian of the foot [stomach meridian] are strong and abundant. If the blood and energy are in abundance in the lower region of the bright yang of the foot meridian, then the pubic hair and the hair on the chest will be long and handsome."

The Chinese believe that a man with plenty of hair on his chest is in possession of strong sexual capability, while a woman with plenty of fine hair on her body is also in possession of strong sexual capability. The man's hair should be of the yang type, firm and strong, while the woman's hair should be of the yin type, soft and smooth.

The number of hairs on the body are roughly estimated at about five million. At first glance, we would say that most of our hair is located on the head, the underarms, and the pubic region. However, fine hairs cover the entire body, at densities similar to those on the more obvious regions. Most hairs are short and fine, so they escape notice, but hairs are present nearly everywhere. And in addition to the millions of hairs on the outside of the body, there are also millions of hairs inside the body; for example, in the ears, in the sweat glands, and lining the digestive tract. (The estimate of five million hairs on the surface of the body is based on information and calculations from *The Human Body: The Essentials of Anatomy and Physiology*, 5th Edition, by Gerard J. Tortora and Sandra Reynolds Grabowski.)

NECK

The neck holds a special place in Chinese sexology. For instance, one method to tonify the breast that can increase the size is to massage the thyroid gland on the neck. According to Chinese medicine, stimulating the sexual organs stimulates the thyroid and vice versa, since the thyroid gland and sexual organs are closely related. When a woman is sexually active, her neck will become longer and expand. Massaging or kissing the woman's neck and thus indirectly the thyroid gland will also stimulate sexual drive.

A large, thick neck on a man indicates strong sexual potential.

BREASTS

According to traditional Chinese medicine, the four parts of the woman's body that reflect her sexuality are her face (that is, eyes and mouth), breasts, buttocks, and vagina. The traditional Chinese sexologists called the breasts "the Bells of Love."

The size of the breasts is only one factor in describing the female sexual capability and potential. The muscles that support the breasts are another factor, because the muscles that support and form the shape of the breasts directly reflect the genitals, since the meridians of the stomach pass through the entire breast area, flowing through the lungs and genitals as well. Through this meridian, one organ gives life to another; it follows that if the muscles that underlie the breast tissue are firm and of good tone, the vaginal muscles will also be firm. Similarly, loose pectoral muscles will indicate a loose vaginal grip.

The Chinese have classified the breasts into groups according to sexual potential.

1. The plate type of breast, or a small-breasted woman, indicates relatively low sexual energy.

2. The bowl type of breast, symmetrical and well-balanced, is shaped like a soup bowl. Each breast is supported by well-toned musculature. This woman will have a high sex drive and is considered the most sexually desirable.

3. The ball type of breast is larger than the bowl type. This woman has even greater sexual energy. When this type of breast includes big nipples and large aureoles, she is sexually powerful.

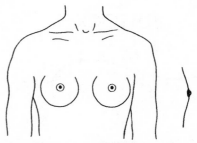

The plate type of breast indicates lower sexual energy

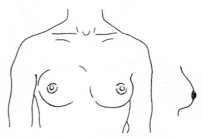

The bowl type of breast indicates a healthy sex drive

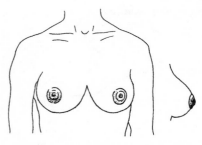

The ball type of breast with large nipples and areolas indicates a very strong and forceful personality

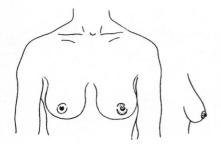

In the pendulum type of breast, if the supporting muscles are strong, this indicates strong sexual potential; if the muscles are flabby, it indicates a weaker sex drive

FEMALE BREAST TYPES

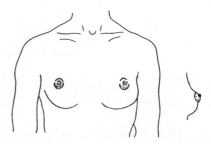

The mountain-peak type of breast is shaped like a peak, with nipples pointing up; this indicates a woman who is very warm and passionate

BUTTOCKS

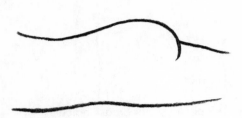

A buttock dipping down indicates strong sexual drive

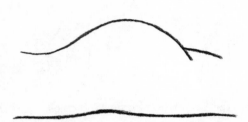

A big buttock indicates a strong, healthy, good wife and mother

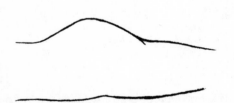

A sharp upper buttock indicates a weak sex drive

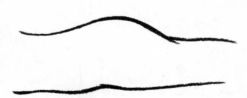

A small buttock with rounding up and down indicates a medium sex drive

BUTTOCKS SIZE AND SHAPE

4. The mountain-peak type of breast is in the shape of a cone with nipples that face the sky. This type of woman is very warm and passionate.

5. The pendulum type of breast is round like a ball hanging from a pendulum. If the muscles supporting this type of breast are solid, this woman's sexual potential is strong. If her muscles are flabby and lack tone, she has a weaker sex drive. If she has no musculature there, as in an older woman, she will have lower sexual energy.

FEMALE BODY

The following points of female beauty are nature's own advertisement of a healthy condition of the sexual system.

1. Large limbs: indicative of strength to sustain the body during the period of pregnancy.

2. Broad hips: indicative of a large pelvis, giving abdominal support during pregnancy and easy delivery.

3. A relatively narrow waist: indicates freedom from suppressed menstruation and a proper expansion of the hips.

Breasts that stand out prominently and are firm in texture, with large nipples free from discoloration surrounded by a bright pink areola, indicate a correct condition of the womb.

A graceful carriage of the body; a springing, vigorous, rhythmical step; sweet breath; good teeth; clear complexion; a pleasant, musical voice; a well-shaped neck and back of the head; red, full lips; a well-developed chin, projecting forward slightly; clear, bright, animated eyes—all are indispensable indications of good sexuality.

The points enumerated in the previous paragraph apply equally well to estimating the sexual strength of the male, with the addition of broad shoulders and a deep chest as well as a contour of body broadest at the shoulders and tapering toward the feet.

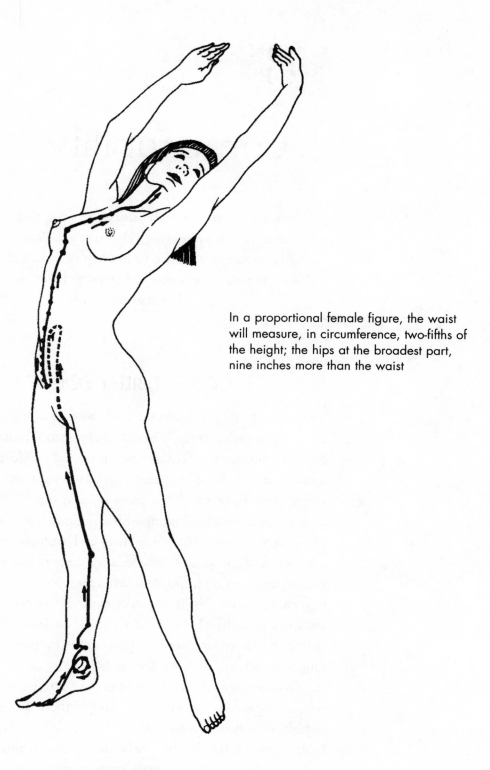

In a proportional female figure, the waist will measure, in circumference, two-fifths of the height; the hips at the broadest part, nine inches more than the waist

FEMALE BODY

Compatibility

When the same inner sight exists in you as in another, you are drawn to be companions. When a man feels in himself the inmost nature of a woman, he is drawn to her sexually. When a woman feels the masculine self of a man within her, she wants him physically in her.

—RUMI

COMPATIBILITY FOR LIFE

The compatibility between men and women offers a glimpse into the unity of the universe. The sexual experience is one of the great gifts of humanity, offering a relatively accessible experience of total balance and harmony and thus serving as a metaphor for the larger purpose of life. That purpose, said the Taoist sages, is to achieve peace and harmony through unification of opposites. Look around you, recognize man and woman as yet another expression of the same cosmic duality that creates day and night, winter and summer, positive and negative, north and south, heaven and earth. Bring together these opposites and the world collapses in spiritual ecstasy, say the Taoist teachers, who regard sex to be as natural and indispensable to human health and longevity as rain falling on the fields.

Compatibility refers to the energetic attraction between two people, especially lovers. Even though there are some obvious indicators of compatibility, or incompatibility, many people overlook them. Compatibility can be determined a number of ways, including through touch, smell, sight, taste, conversation, holding hands, interest, chemistry, and energy.

Compatibility should be like a good red wine, becoming richer and deeper over time. This is why relationships should be given ample time in each stage of progression: courting, dating, and marriage. With the Taoist secrets of love techniques, a relationship gets more profound and intense the longer you stay with your partner. This is because the Taoists learn to cultivate energy rather than drain it. If a couple who have deep affection and love for one another drain each other's energy through sexual indulgence, emotional ups and downs, and needless arguments, the intensity and depth of the relationship diminishes. This is one of the reasons for such a high divorce rate in the West. With the Taoist techniques, love grows and flourishes.

In the West, compatibility is sometimes referred to as chemistry. When a couple has "good chemistry," there is electrical, magnetic energy. The age-old question is how to keep this magnetism, this chemistry with partners so that it will last a lifetime. The Taoists discovered this secret in the cultivation of energy. When there is energy in a relationship, there is interest, excitement, and joy.

The Taoists view compatibility from a variety of perspectives. One way compatibility can be revealed is through the sense of smell. Smell is one of the primal senses of attraction, both consciously and subconsciously. In some cultures, smelling the neck and the face is just as erotic as passionately kissing. We can use the sense of smell to determine whether we are compatible with someone. If a partner's scent is revolting, you might want to reassess the relationship. This does not mean smelling your partner after a three-hour workout; it means the partner's smell in general. Is it pleasant to the nose when you are holding each other close, when you are kissing or snuggling?

There are many other ways to determine the compatibility of men and women. For example, when you clasp hands with a partner, note the harmony or disharmony of the clasp itself. If the hands do not seem to fit harmoniously and if the contact becomes unpleasant when prolonged, it is a sure sign that the dispositions will not harmonize. If the clasp is harmonious and the effect of prolonged contact continues to be agreeable, it indicates that the general effect is harmonious.

In every intimate association, kisses and caresses will provide the most important information. Caresses and kisses must be

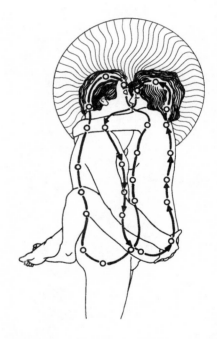

FUSION OF THE MICROCOSMIC ORBITS

exchanged with great freedom, and the kisses must be sufficiently passionate and complete to enable the couple to obtain the full effect of the flavor of the fluid and the magnetic or electric effect of the caresses. If the caresses exert a highly beneficial effect and the kisses increase in sweetness and enjoyment over time, it is a good indicator of growth potential. If this result is not reached and the kisses become repulsive and the caresses become weak or the parties find after complete and intimate association that love does not continually augment in intensity, the conditions of harmony are absent and all thought of continued companionship should be dismissed. However, the parties may continue to be affectionate friends as long as it is mutually agreeable. This judgment should not be formed hastily, and I consider it unsafe to form a conclusion from any impression that may be only momentary. I recommend that this experiment, taking the time to just be friends, last at least six months, unless the parties discover in a shorter time that it is positively disagreeable. In some of the best adaptations I have known, it took some time for the best results to be established, especially in those cases where the parties were young and inexperienced and had not learned the art of expressing their emotions freely. Love, like everything else, is a creature of growth and takes time to develop.

Waiting or postponing sexual intercourse allows the heart to be seasoned with love. Sexual intercourse that occurs too soon drains energy, especially if one is not skilled at the Taoist arts of the bedchamber. Promiscuity has a tendency to prevent this energy from cultivating in the heart center.

When walking together with a partner, keep in step and notice if it is an easy thing to do and if the gait of one is harmonious with the other. The walk is an unfailing indication of character, and it is impossible for persons who experience great difficulty in keeping step or who tire each other when walking together to harmonize in character.

Notice the effect of conversation. If after a long conversation you experience a feeling of fatigue and you find this the usual result, the partner's character is inharmonious with your own. Language is the principal avenue of expression, and its effects cannot be too closely watched. If the conversation inspires you and you feel rested and instructed after each occasion, or this is generally the result, the indications are in favor of harmony. Many couples fall in love or notice the attractive energy first from conversation.

Some cultures are sufficiently well informed to know the desirability of preliminary tests of intimate association before marriage, and the custom of "bundling" among the Dutch and similar customs among other nationalities have their origin in a crude effort to establish a test of this kind. In the custom of bundling, the male and female are each sewed up in a sack in such a manner that it is impossible to have sexual intercourse without rupturing the sacks and thus being detected. In this condition they are allowed to sleep together and note the effect upon their feelings. Whatever may be the general result of such a practice, there is no question as to its value as a test. It is impossible for two persons to sleep together a number of nights without becoming conscious either of increased affection and desire for companionship or of the entire loss of such desire. The effect of sleeping together may be summed up as follows: If the parties are not harmonious, they will in a short time exhaust their magnetism to such a degree that all mutual attraction ceases. If they are harmonious, the effect will be delightful and the desire for its continuance will increase for a number of months. Then there will be a culmination in which no great degree of increased desire will be felt, but it will continue to be a pleasant experience. If the parties are perfectly harmonious, this may continue for many years, but as a general rule the pleasure of contact will be greatly intensified if they do not continually sleep together. If they are not perfectly harmonious, the magnetism will gradually be lost; hence, as very few couples are perfectly harmonious, it is a good rule to occupy separate beds and sleep together only occasionally as desired and as expediency may dictate. The loss of magnetism, and the consequent neutralizing of affection, will be slow or rapid in its progress as the parties are more or less harmonious.

The period of experimental courtship (intimate physical contact that excludes sexual intercourse) may be as long or short as the prudence and the circumstances of the parties may dictate, but I suggest that six months is not unreasonably long, and I also believe that any reasonable man or woman ought to be thoroughly satisfied with the results of such a test in one year of continued intimate association.

LOVEMAKING ENERGY

Do you not see that you and I are as the branches of one tree?
With your rejoicing comes my laughter; with your sadness
start my tears.
Love, could life be otherwise with you and me?

—Tsu Yeh Tsin dynasty, a.d. 265–316

The following exercise will balance and harmonize the male and female energies of the partners. The Tao calls this exercise energetic lovemaking.

Sit cross-legged facing your partner. The woman places her hands palms up on her knees; the man places his palms face down in hers so that the centers of the palms touch.

Take some long, slow, deep breaths, breathing in unison and synchronizing the inhale and exhale. This synchronizes the energy between each other. Feel the exchange of energy flowing between the palms. You can visualize a god and goddess above your head making love. Feel the energy pouring down onto the crown of the head and into the whole body. Feel the sexual energy of the universe in harmony with your own sexual energy. Allow the intimate connection between yourself, your partner, and the universe to pulse through your entire being.

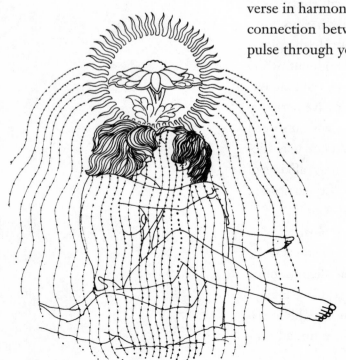

Visualizing the sexual energy of the universe

Sexercises

In the Tao, sexual exercises were not merely a way to enhance sexual pleasure or become more attractive. These exercises were a means to enjoy a more vigorous and healthy body, a way to become sensitive to deeper and more intense emotions and to cultivate spiritual energy. The Taoists believed that the body would stay healthy and youthful as long as it was able to reproduce. When the reproductive energy was in a decline, the body would retaliate with sickness or emotional insecurity.

In the East as well as in the West, exercise is a crucial way to keep the body healthy. But when it comes to increasing sexual energy, the teachers of the East have taken exercise to a higher level. To strengthen our sexual energy and thus strengthen the senses and the whole body, the Eastern traditions have developed exercises that focus specifically on the sexual area.

By strengthening the sexual organs through exercise and massage, we actually affect the rest of the body and senses. It is believed that the sexual organs are the strongest reflex points in the body and when stimulated in the proper way can have a powerful healing effect on the senses and internal organs, making you healthier and more sexy. There are pelvic exercises that greatly strengthen the reproductive organs and the complex network of tendons in the surrounding area. Strength in this department is of great importance; it is the root of both a man's and a woman's health. Leading into the pelvis are a vast number of nerve endings and channels for the veins and arteries. Here are located tissues that communicate with every square inch of the body. All the major acupuncture meridians that carry energy between the body and the vital organs pass by this area. If it is blocked or weak, energy will dissipate and the organs and brain will suffer. These

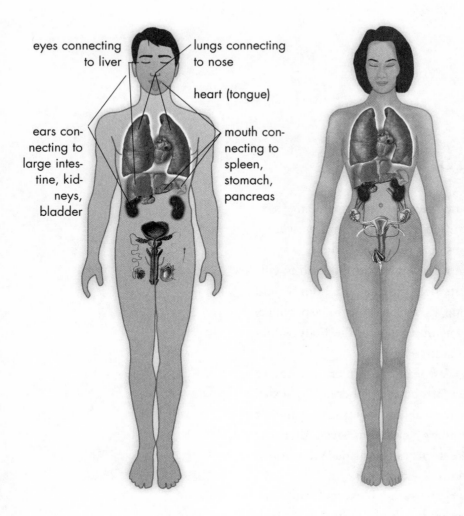

exercises are designed to charge the brain with energy, increase circulation, stimulate nerve flow, strengthen the urogenital diaphragm, and tonify the energy of the sexual organs. Because they focus on enhancing the strength and energy of the sexual area, we have called this workout "sexercises."

In the Taoist view of sexual health, it is important to cultivate our sexual energy rather than needlessly wasting it. For men this means regulating and controlling ejaculation. For women it means working with and balancing the female menstruation cycle.

If men ejaculate too often, it depletes the source of vital energy, not allowing the water of life to spread to the rest of the body. The importance of a man's retaining semen is em-

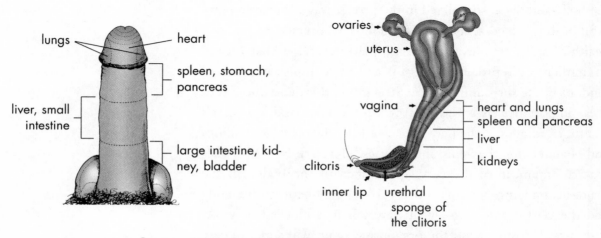

SEXUAL REFLEXOLOGY POINTS THROUGHOUT THE BODY

phasized over and over again in Taoist literature, which is dramatically different from the religious idea of celibacy. In the Tao, regulating and managing ejaculation does not mean becoming a celibate. The basic purpose of these methods is to increase, as much as possible, the quantity of the life-giving, age-retarding hormones secreted in a man's body during sexual excitement while at the same time decreasing, as much as possible, the loss of semen and its related hormones through ejaculation. All schools of Taoism agree that semen retention and proper regulation of its emission are indispensable skills for male adepts. To understand more about this concept, I recommend reading *The Multi-Orgasmic Man* by Mantak Chia and Douglas Abram and *Taoist Secrets of Love* by Mantak Chia.

BREATHING SEXERCISES

There is one way of breathing that is shameful and constricted.
Then there's another way: a breath of love that takes you
all the way to infinity.

—RUMI, *OPEN SECRET*

The first step to becoming a more sexually powerful person is to learn how to breathe properly. Many of the sexercises require a certain level of breath control, and when you learn to breathe properly, the exercises become much easier and much more powerful. Breathing exercises are a direct way to control stress.

For example, think about how you breathe when you are in a terribly stressful situation. The breath gets jammed up in the chest in short, shallow gasps that barely allow oxygen into the lungs. Under extreme circumstances the breath might become almost nonexistent. With this type of breathing, life-enhancing oxygen does not flow freely through the body. This creates stress and tension, lodging it in the body rather than allowing it to be processed and released.

Long ago in Chinese medicine it was discovered that the breath is a direct reflection of the emotional state of the body. When someone is sad, the person breathes in short, inhaling gasps, locking the air in the upper chest. When someone is angry, the breath is usually long, contracted exhales, with desperately short inhalations. Even when we are not feeling very emotional, the breath will still reflect the general overall feelings in the body, which are often not very empowering.

Just as correct diet enhances the body's store of nutritional essence, so correct breathing enhances the body's supply of vital energy. Proper breathing is performed by the diaphragm, not the rib cage and the clavicles. Because of laziness, ignorance, smoking, pollution, constipation, and other factors, adults these days invariably become shallow chest breathers rather than the deep abdominal breathers that we are meant to be. All true martial arts and meditation practices use the breath as the gate to control the body.

Breathing abdominally is the most natural thing; it is just that we have forgotten how we used to breathe. Have you ever watched a baby breathe? Notice how the stomach or abdomen does the breathing, not the chest. This is the natural way, the way we have to return to.

Chest breathing employs the intercostal muscles between the ribs to forcibly expand the upper rib cage, thereby lowering air pressure in the chest so that air enters by suction. However, this leaves the lower lungs, which contain by far the greatest surface area, immobilized. Consequently one must take about three times as many chest breaths in order to get the same quantity of air into the lungs as provided by a single diaphragmatic breath.

Deep Abdominal Breathing (for Men and Women)

A complete, deep, abdominal breath should employ three areas of the lungs in a smooth, unbroken expansion that begins at the bottom, in the abdomen, and not in the upper chest. One first inhales air slowly into the lower lungs by letting the diaphragm expand and balloon downward into the abdominal cavity. When the diaphragm is fully expanded, the intercostal muscles come into play to open the rib cage and fill the middle lungs with air. As the rib cage reaches full expansion, the breather utilizes the clavicles so that air flows into the narrow upper pockets of the lungs.

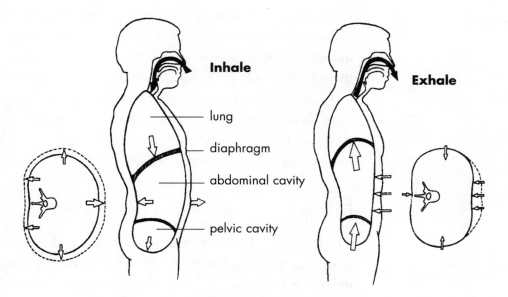

Inhale

Exhale

- lung
- diaphragm
- abdominal cavity
- pelvic cavity

DEEP ABDOMINAL BREATHING

Exhale in the reverse manner, releasing air from the upper part of the chest, downward through the ribs, finally expelling the air out the lower lungs by slightly contracting the abdomen. Breathing with the diaphragm in this manner reduces the number of breaths per minute by more than half, greatly enhances respiratory efficiency, saves the heart from strain, and conserves vital energy.

This type of breathing has many benefits for the body and emotions. When we are able to breathe in this manner, the body automatically takes it as a sign to be relaxed and calm. This is one of the best ways to combat the stress of everyday life. If you can, practice deep abdominal breathing whenever you have a few extra minutes, driving the car, standing in line, waiting for the dentist, or anywhere else you can imagine; great benefits will result. With practice, your body will soon automatically start breathing deeper without conscious intention.

Deep abdominal breathing activates the cranial and sacral pumps, movement of minute bone structures that keep the spinal fluid moving in the joints and cranium. Spinal fluid and seminal fluid are very similar in nature.

Deep abdominal breathing is a wonderful exercise for increasing sexual energy. It sends energy down through the urogenital diaphragm, loosening and relaxing the whole pelvic cavity.

Without deep breathing, the lower abdomen has a tendency to become tight and contracted. This leads to low sexual energy or uncontrollable sexual energy. With this tightness in the abdomen, there is inevitably an imbalance throughout the sexual area. For men, tightness can cause premature ejaculation, nocturnal emissions, impotence, or sexual frustration. For women, this tightness can cause menstrual cramps, frigid sexual energy, PMS, and other more complicated emotional problems.

Energy Breathing (for Men and Women)

The energy breath is performed by rapidly expelling air out of the lungs and is designed to create efficient circulation, strengthening the energy of the lower abdominal area. Imagine that there is a small fire right behind the navel. To build this small spark into a vibrant fire requires air. As you perform the exercise, the breath should sound like a bellows fanning a fire. Start by forcefully expelling all air from the lungs with a strong contraction of the abdominal wall. Immediately after the expulsion of air, let the lungs fill naturally without effort, about halfway. When the lungs are half full, immediately contract the abdominal wall again to forcefully expel another gust of air. The exercise should consist of about twenty to thirty rapid expulsions of air. This strengthens and energizes the lower abdominal area (Sexual Palace and Lower Tan Tien).

SEXERCISE MASSAGES

Massage is a great way to get in touch with our bodies. It has been used for thousands of years as a way to achieve health, relaxation, and longevity. The reason massage is so beneficial is that it releases pent-up tension caused by stress and establishes communication between the mind and the body. By increasing circulation, releasing muscle adhesions, and generating positive energy, massage is of utmost importance.

Throughout the book we have discussed ways to massage the body to increase energy in the sexual center. Now we discuss massaging the sexual center itself, not only to enhance sexual energy but to increase the energy in the whole body.

Testicle Massage

Testicle massage is a way to connect consciously to the male sexual energy. It is critically important to differentiate these exercises from masturbation. In the Tao, the goal of the practice is to harness this vital energy, not to release it. It is essential that you feel the energy and bring it up into the whole body.

Begin by sitting on the edge of a chair, without trousers or underclothing. (It is possible to do this exercise while wearing pants, but it is important that they be loose so that the material does not interfere with the massage. It is a good idea to always wear pants that do not constrict the blood flow to the genitals. In general, it is always better to wear loose rather than tight pants and underwear.)

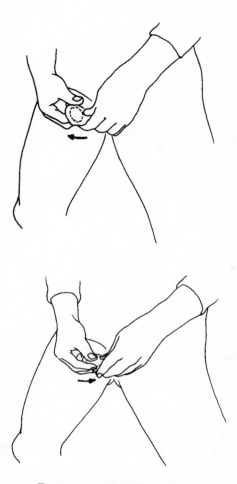

ROLLING TESTICLE MASSAGE

Rolling Testicle Massage ❖ Rub your palms together till warm, then place the tips of all four fingers underneath the testicles, with thumbs on top, and massage the testicles firmly by rolling them around between fingertips and thumbs. Roll the testicles about thirty-six times in each direction. Perform a few PC muscle contractions, and finish with deep abdominal breathing.

This exercise increases the production of testosterone, sperm, and seminal fluids and elevates male sexual energy in a powerful yet balanced way.

The testicles are the most important part of the reproductive organs because they hold the key to developing testosterone and sperm. If you neglect them, then you will not be able to perform sexually as you desire. The increased production of testosterone that results from testicle massage in turn raises your drive for sex. These exercises also promote better blood circulation to your testicles, increasing sperm count and ejaculation volume.

The testicles are vital organs in the body, and without them we would be an extinct species. Keeping them in shape will not only give you harder erections, more sex drive, and greater amounts of semen but will also give you a healthier sperm count and a better chance for conception when you try to have children. The key to proper testicle function and health is better blood circulation to your testicles.

Testicle Circulation Massage ❀ Massage between your testicles with a pumping motion, using your thumb and fingers. Massage at the base, pulling it down as you massage. Do this for about three minutes. Take your hands with your fingers spread apart and grip your testicles at the root and lightly pull them down, bring them back up, them pull them down again, over and over for about three minutes. Lightly apply pressure to your testicles, massaging them while doing so. Massage all around them, working your way around both of the testicles. Continue to repeat all of these steps over and over again. This massaging routine should be done for at least ten minutes a day, preferably in the morning or before bedtime.

Three times a week you should stretch out your testicle skin really well, feeling a good stretch as you pull the skin down. Grasp around the base of your testicles with your thumb and forefinger and squeeze until your testicles are tight together on top of your thumb and forefinger. Take the other hand and apply a small amount of pressure on top of the testicles and massage them in a circular motion. While you are doing this, pull down lightly with the hand grasping the base of your testicles. Do this for about three to five minutes without stopping.

After these massaging exercises, your testicles should be stretched out and appear to be hanging lower than normal. They should also appear to be larger. This is due to the increased blood circulated into your testicles from performing these exercises. You should do these massaging and stretching techniques at least three to four times a week, but daily exercise can be performed for absolute optimal testicle health and fertility. The heat generated will increase the blood flow as well as allowing the essence to be absorbed back into your body more quickly.

TESTICLE CIRCULATION MASSAGE

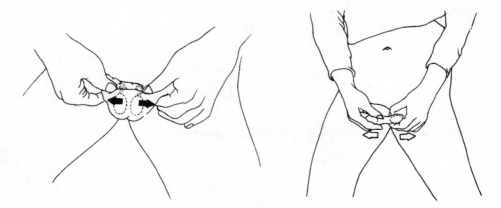

Tapping the Dragon Pearls (for Men)

By tapping on the testicles one can directly stimulate the kidney energy of the body. Remember, the kidneys govern the sexual energy. Tapping the testicles stimulates hormonal production through the entire endocrine system.

Stand in a wide stance or sit on the edge of a chair. Rub your palms together until warm, then use one hand to grasp the penis and pull it upward. The fingertips of the other hand gently tap the testicles so that they bounce up and down. Do not tap so hard that it is painful, but hard enough to feel it all over the lower abdomen. Do about thirty-six taps with each hand. After tapping, contract and relax the PC muscle. Follow this with some deep breathing.

Penis Power Stretching

To achieve optimal results by stretching your penis, you must understand how the penis works. The penis is made up of cells that enlarge when they fill with blood. These cells are called blood spaces. The blood spaces are within your erectile tissue, also known as the corpora cavernosa. When you stretch the penis, you are stretching all parts of the penis, including the areas that fill with blood. When these areas have stretched to a certain length, the penis will extend longer in both the flaccid and erect state. What most people do not understand is that the penis is probably the easiest part of your body to lengthen and thicken because of the simple fact of its anatomy. The erection is the size it is because the cells within the penis are a certain size. By naturally causing blood to fill the spaces through exercising, or by stretching the flesh, penis enlargement is quite possible with minimal effort.

1. Inhale fully; now exhale and flatten the abdomen while sticking the tongue out. Use the thumb and index finger to grip the head of the penis, resting the other hand at the base. Pull the penis and thrust the tongue out more. Keep on pulling until you need to inhale. Gasp the air into the intestines; exhale making a *shhhhh* sound until out of breath. Do this step a few times before moving on to step 2.

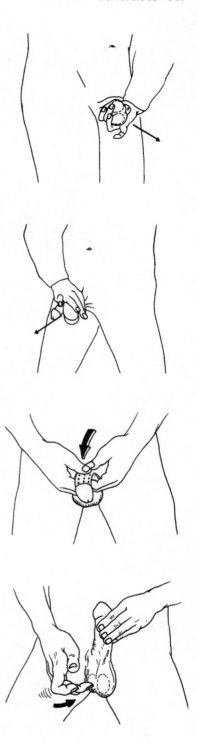

TESTICLE MASSAGE AND TESTICLE TAPPING

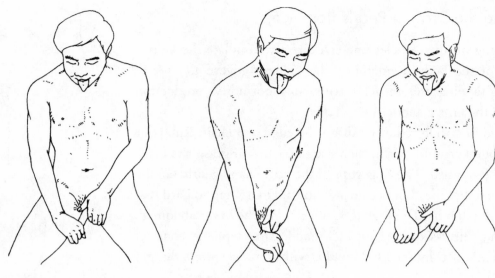

POWER STRETCHING

2. In a standing or sitting position, make sure the penis is in a completely flaccid state and grasp around the head, not so tight as to cause pain but just to ensure a good grip.

3. Pull the penis directly out in front of you until you feel a good stretch in the middle and at the base. Hold this stretch for a count of ten, then rest and feel the energy from the sexual organs. Repeat three more times.

4. Now slap your penis against the leg about fifty times to get the blood back into the area you have been squeezing.

5. Next, grasp around the penis again; exhale, sticking out the tongue. This time pull to your far left until you feel a good stretch on the right side at the base. Hold this position for a count of ten and repeat. Rest and guide the sexual energy to the crown.

6. Slap the penis against the leg fifty times again.

7. Grasp around the penis, sticking out the tongue and holding the breath, only this time pull to your far right until you feel a good stretch on the left side at the base. Hold this position for a count of ten. Repeat three more times.

8. Slap the penis against the leg fifty times again.

Rotations

1. Grasp around the penis's head and pull outward until you feel a good stretch.

2. Once extended, begin by rotating the penis in a circular fashion to your left—not twisting, but rotating in a circular motion. You should feel a good stretch from all areas of the penis and at the base where it connects. Do thirty rotations, then rest for a few seconds and gently contract the anus and perineum, guiding the Chi up to the crown. Then repeat three more times.

3. Slap the penis against your leg fifty times to get the blood flowing again.

4. Repeat step 2, this time rotating the penis to the right. Do the same rotation technique as before, only this time to your right. Do thirty rotations.

5. Rest for a few seconds, then repeat entire exercise three more times.

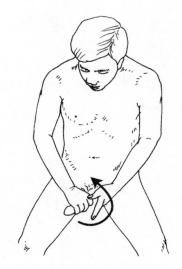

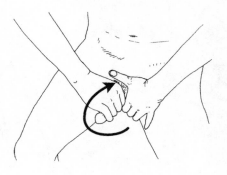

ROTATIONS

Hot Hands Warm-Up

The purpose in Taoist penis enlargement is to enlarge the corpora cavernosa, the spongy tissue that fills with blood when you get an erection. Just as you should warm up your body and muscle tissue before any workout, you should do the same for your penis. This will prepare it for the workout ahead by making the blood spaces in the corpora cavernosa hot, which expands the tissue and makes it more flexible and spongy. If you start out performing the exercises cold, you are more likely to experience bruising or goose bumps than you would if you prepared your penis for the physical workout it is about to undergo. The following exercise, called the Hot Hands Warm-Up, should be done before and after every workout you do to your penis and testicles.

1. Rub your hands warm.

2. Hold the penis between the two palms and rub until warm.

3. Hold the testicles between the palms and rub them warm.

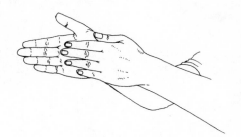

RUB HANDS

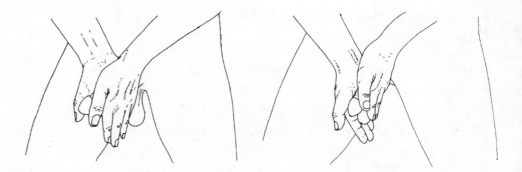

PENIS AND TESTICLE WARM-UP

Vaginal Stretch

As for women, use the same procedure with the egg with a string to lengthen and strengthen the vagina canal. Squeeze the egg and pull the string. Keep on pulling until you need to inhale. Gasp the air into the intestines; exhale making a *shhhhh* sound until you are out of breath.

USE VISUALIZATION TO INCREASE SEXUAL ENERGY

The more you foresee your results and the more you focus on where you want to be, the faster you will get there. As you perform the following exercises, take care and always remember to visualize your goals. Visualize the Microcosmic Orbit movement and fill the organs with Chi. Really focus on your penis; close your eyes and get a good picture in your mind as you exercise. Now, in the upcoming exercises, every time you milk, stretch, or PC flex, visualize your penis and pineal gland growing a little bit each time and becoming the size that you desire. Focus on every stroke you take, and as you stretch, simultaneously visualize a good stretch. Focus on the size you want to be and visualize that you have already achieved this. The more you make visualization a regular part of your penile fitness workout, the faster and better results you will attain. This concept goes for anything you do, whether it is penile fitness, exercise, body conditioning, or meditation. Keeping yourself in top physical shape is very important to your health. Prostate

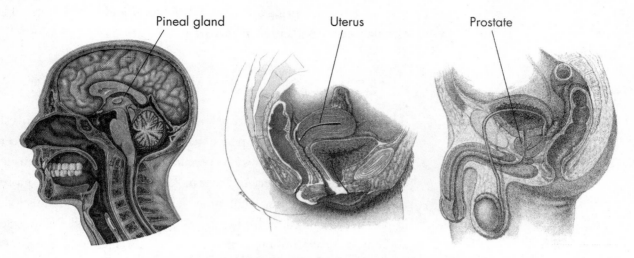

Pineal gland   Uterus   Prostate

CENTER OF THE BRAIN CONNECTS TO THE SEXUAL ORGANS

disease and cancer are a leading cause of death in males over the age of fifty, and with worsening health conditions each year, it's important that you take responsibility for your own health.

SEXUAL ORGANS AND THE BRAIN

The sexual organs (ovaries, testicles, uterus, prostate gland) have a close connection to the center of the brain, especially the pineal gland. Circulating the sexual energy down to the sacrum and then up to the brain will increase the brain memory. The Taoist sage says, "Return the sexual energy to revitalize the brain."

The center of the brain is connected to the uterus and prostate gland. Contracting and

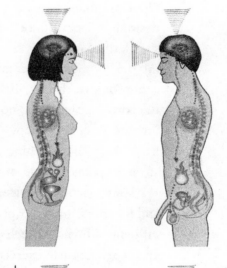

Changing the physical (sperm and eggs) to etheric and the material to immaterial

DRAWING THE SEXUAL ENERGY UP TO THE BRAIN

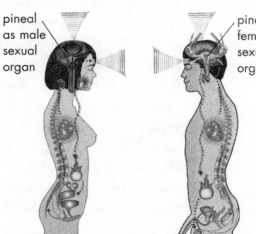

pineal as male sexual organ

pineal as female sexual organ

In women the pineal is the male sexual organ, and in men the pineal is the female sexual organ.

PINEAL GLAND IS THE SECOND SEXUAL ORGAN

releasing the sex organs increases the blood and sexual hormone circulation to the center of the brain.

PC MUSCLE AND MILKING EXERCISES

The PC muscle and milking exercises stretch out the central tendon-like tissue in your penis, making it longer while both erect and flaccid. These exercises also promote an increase in testosterone and sperm count. It's very sad that in America alone there are more than thirty million impotent men. This is horrifying because all impotence is caused by having a weak, underdeveloped PC muscle and corpora cavernosa (erectile tissue). If you have weak erections or have bouts of impotence regularly, this means that you have very poor blood circulation to your penis and testicles. Having proper blood circulation to any part of your body is vital if good health is desired. A lack of blood circulation to the penis will weaken and shrink the corpora cavernosa and also lessen the sensation and feeling during intercourse, hence promoting impotence. The milking action of stretching will force blood into the blood spaces within the corpora cavernosa, not only enlarging the penis but also training the body to accept more blood flow throughout the entire penis. Regular stretching will ensure a well-circulated, healthy, and stronger penis after several months of vigorous exercise.

Your ejaculatory strength and ability, your erectile strength and firmness, and your prostate health and wellness are all directly influenced by how much you perform the PC muscle and milking exercises. Regular exercise will greatly develop your PC muscle, which in turn will give you hard erections, improve blood circulation to the penis, substantially increase ejaculation volume and intensity, and actually give you a very healthy prostate. This will help prevent prostate cancer, a leading cause of death in men. The squeeze and flex exercises are simply an advanced PC (pubococcygeus) muscle exercise that incorporates a medium to a tight grip around the erect penis as you perform. This adds resistance to your PC workout by squeezing against the pulsating erection as you flex your PC muscle. Many months of PC Chi muscle exercise is needed for the average man to be able to last very long in lovemaking.

As you flex the PC muscle, contract the eyes, mouth, anus, and prostate gland. This will activate the center of the brain.

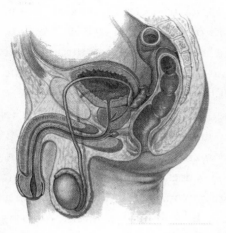
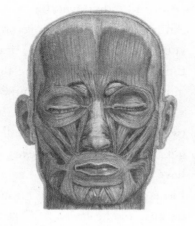
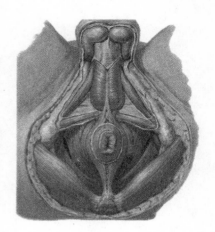

PELVIC VISCERA AND PERINEUM OF MALE

CHI MUSCLE

When you exercise your PC muscle, also called Chi muscle, you will develop ejaculatory control, which will prevent the premature urge to ejaculate. You will also improve blood circulation for enhanced size and sensation, greatly improve sexual stamina, and improve urinary flow and the ability to have multiple orgasms.

The first step to beginning your PC workout is locating your PC muscle. Some men have been able to locate their PC muscle for

MALE PELVIC AND UROGENITAL DIAPHRAGMS

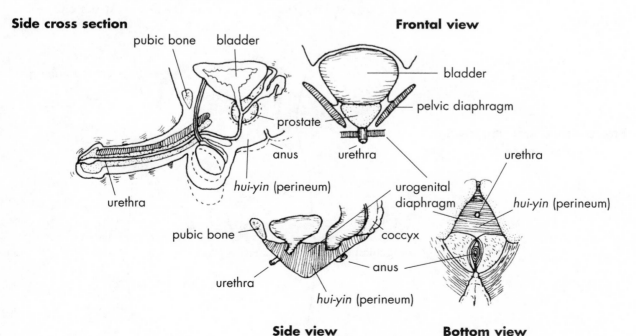

Side cross section

pubic bone   bladder

prostate

anus

hui-yin (perineum)

urethra

Frontal view

bladder

pelvic diaphragm

urethra

pubic bone

urethra

hui-yin (perineum)

Side view

urogenital diaphragm

coccyx

anus

urethra

hui-yin (perineum)

Bottom view

years and didn't even know it. Quick test: Get an erection. If you can make your penis move on its own when you have an erection, you have located your PC muscle. If you cannot do this, the next time you urinate, stop the flow of urine before you finish. The muscle you use to stop yourself from urinating is the PC muscle.

Once you have located the PC muscle, continue with ten to twenty flexes to see how well you can focus on them. If your PC gets tired after twenty flexes, you are very out of shape. After you have done twenty or so, flex and squeeze really tightly and hold it for as long as you can. Though this may be intimidating at first because of the lack of PC strength, within a few months of continual exercise, men will be able to hold off the urge to ejaculate just by squeezing the PC muscle as tight as they can until the urge passes.

Men and women can enhance their sexual prowess and energy by doing at least two hundred to five hundred PC flexes a day. Ancient Taoists also called the exercise "tightening the anus" because it also makes your anus tight when you flex.

PC CHI MUSCLE EXERCISES

Warming Up ❖ Start out by squeezing and relaxing the PC muscle at a steady pace for a good thirty flexes. At the end of the

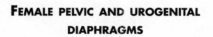

FEMALE PELVIC AND UROGENITAL DIAPHRAGMS

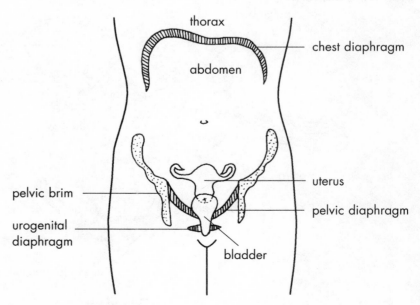

set, rest for thirty seconds. Continue with two more sets, resting for thirty seconds between each set. After this is complete, you should have better control over your PC muscle owing to the increased blood and Chi flow.

PC Clamps ◈ Squeeze and release the PC muscle over and over again. Start with sets of thirty, and build yourself up to a set of one hundred or more. The PC muscle recovers quite quickly from any soreness, and you may find yourself waking up with a hard erection every morning. Make sure you do at least three hundred PC clamps a day for the rest of your life. You will soon find that it's the best move you could make for your sexual health and vitality.

Long Slow Squeeze ◈ Warm up with a set of thirty PC muscle clamps, then flex as hard and as deep as you possibly can. When you cannot squeeze any deeper, hold where you are for a twenty count. Rest for thirty seconds. Repeat five times. After a month or so of exercising, you should be able to do squeeze-and-hold sessions for at least several minutes at a time. This particular exercise will give you erections of absolute steel and the ability to prolong lovemaking as long as you want. Eventually work your way up to ten sets of two-minute holds.

PC Steps Workout ◈ In this exercise you simply tighten and loosen your PC muscle in increments. Begin to tighten your PC, hold, then tighten more, hold, a little more, hold, then tighten as much as you possibly can and hold. Hold this for twenty seconds, then release a little bit, hold, release a little bit more, hold, a little more, hold, then finally release the rest. Do this five times with no rest in between.

TESTICLE STRETCHING EXERCISE

Testicle stretching is an important part of the PC muscle training program.

1. Warm up as you did for PC exercises.

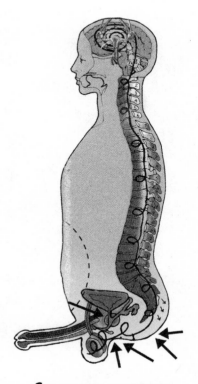

CHI MUSCLE SQUEEZING

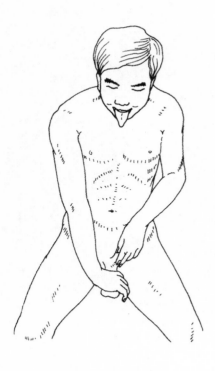

2. Grasp around the testicles with one hand and the penis with the other and begin stretching them in opposite directions, up and down, and exhaling while flattening the stomach and sticking out the tongue. Stop when you feel a good stretch and hold for twenty seconds.

3. After the twenty seconds, relax for a few seconds and grasp around your testicles and penis again.

4. Stretch again, only this time pulling your testicles to the left and your penis to your right. Feel a good stretch and hold for twenty seconds. Rest for ten seconds.

5. Stretch again, only this time pulling your testicles to the right and your penis to your left. Wait until you feel a good stretch and hold for twenty seconds. Rest for ten seconds.

6. Stretch again, only this time pulling your testicles down and your penis up. Wait until you feel a good stretch and hold for thirty seconds.

POWER MILKING

Power Milking is more of a penis enlargement exercise, but it has many beneficial penile-health-inducing properties when done regularly. The tongue is an important part of the exercise because it is connected to all the tendons of the body, especially the penis, which consists of many tendons. When milking, stick the tongue out, and the tongue will get longer as well as the penis.

It is recommended that you use a lubricant when performing the following exercise. Your choice for lubrication is a crucial one, because if you choose a lubricant that evaporates easily, then you will get tired of reapplying it. You can use baby oil with Vitamin E. It is a good lubricant for exercise, plus it is also nice to apply to the penis and testicles after showering, to keep them healthy and supple.

Men should always start out by stretching out the penis lightly by grasping around the head, sticking out the tongue, and pulling outward. Rotate the tongue as you rotate your penis outward in a circular motion.

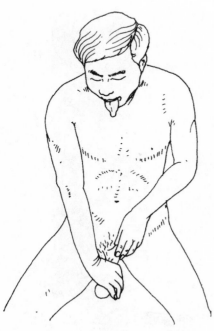

TESTICLE STRETCHING

When warming up has been completed, proceed with the milking method.

1. Lightly massage the penis to a partial erection to hold blood within its length.

2. Grasp around the base (bottom) of the penis shaft with the thumb and forefinger of one hand. This retains the blood within the penis. With the other hand grasp all the way around the penis, making an "OK" sign with the forefinger and thumb, and grip tightly.

3. With your thumb and forefinger squeezed all the way around your penis, slide them forward slowly, taking three to four seconds. This forces the blood within the penis forward into the corpora cavernosa (erectile tissue) and the glans (head).

4. The blood spaces within the penis are forced to expand every time you milk forward. As one hand milks forward to the beginning of the head, grasp around the base of the shaft with the other hand, releasing the hand that has reached the head, and repeat with the other hand, over and over again at a medium to slow pace (one-second intervals).

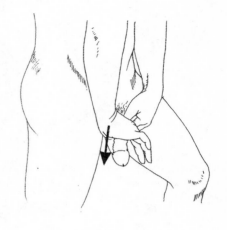

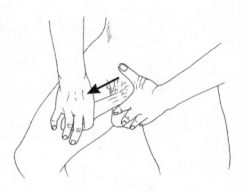

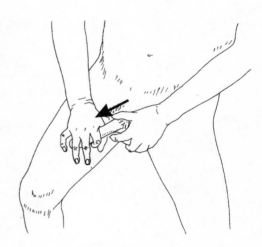

POWER MILKING

When first starting the milking, some men experience red spots, bumps, or light bruising on the penis head and surrounding areas. Don't worry; this is perfectly normal and will usually subside within the first week of exercise. These effects are simply caused by the stretching of the blood spaces within your penis and the new increased blood circulation.

In the beginning, start out by doing three hundred milks (five minutes) a day. Follow this by warming the area with your hands for fifteen minutes. Each milking should last three to four seconds from grasping the base and sliding to the head. Do this for one week and be sure to do one hundred PC flexes a day in addition. This will aid in the new circulation and strength building taking place within your penis.

The second week will be much harder than the first: ten minutes of continuous milking, followed by two hundred PC Chi muscle flexes. Do not ease up unless you happen to feel pain, though this is highly unlikely. Apply a rub for ten minutes to finish the session.

If the continuous exercise forms painful bruising on the penis, stop all exercising and wait for the bruising to subside. You can always perform PC flexes and stretching; get into the habit of doing PC flexes while driving or sitting at work, school, or elsewhere. PC flexes are so important to the overall development and health of the penis.

MILKING AND HOLDING

The milk-and-hold technique is something men should incorporate after first milking for at least twenty minutes. This makes the penis and all the spongy tissue within the penis warmed up and stretched out enough that the chance of injury due to overexertion is very minimal. This exercise thickens and lengthens the penis in both its erect and flaccid state.

Warming Up ◈ Massage the penis to an erection and flex the PC muscle to make it as hard as possible. Once fully erect, pump the PC twenty times to expand the penis as much as possible. Squeeze the PC as hard as you can and hold until the erection reduces somewhat. Now it is time to milk.

Milking ◈ Apply the choice of lubricant and begin the method of milking. While you milk, visualize the penis lengthening each time you milk down to the head. Milk for twenty minutes continuously without stopping. Once completed, rest for a minute and keep massaging your penis to keep it in a partially erect state. Now you are ready for the milk and hold.

Milk and Hold ◈ Begin milking just as you have been, but perform each milk with about a two-second interval. Now, after about twenty milks, milk down a little harder than normal. If you are doing it firmly, the hand should stop when it comes to the head. When this happens, pull hard enough to feel a good stretch in the penis. Repeat the twenty-milk set, then perform the milk-and-hold with the opposite hand. Continue with this routine over and over again for a total of five hundred milkings and twenty-five milk-and-holds.

Cooling Down ◈ At the end of this workout the penis should feel very fatigued and appear quite "pumped" or full-looking. Massage the penis to a full, hard erection and flex the PC muscle several times while massaging to enlarge the penis to its fullest potential. Keep massaging and pumping the PC until the urge to ejaculate is quite strong. Once this sensation is reached, flex the PC as hard as possible, cutting off any possibility of semen's passing through the ejaculatory duct. Keep flexing until the urge is gone, then repeat. Do this five times to cool down.

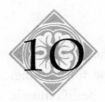

Internal Organs and the Five Elements

The Five Elemental Energies of Wood, Fire, Earth, Metal and Water encompass all the myriad phenomena of nature. It is a paradigm that applies equally to humans.

—THE YELLOW EMPEROR'S CLASSIC OF INTERNAL MEDICINE

(SECOND CENTURY B.C.E.)

Sexual prowess, as one aspect of human compatibility and behavior, is derived from the strength of the internal organs. In order to determine by observation a person's sexual potential, it is necessary to know the person's internal-organ energy levels. Using the information derived from sexual reflexology, a simple examination of the person's physiognomy can reveal his or her character or disposition and will help you to determine the nature of the individual. These principles can also help you better understand your own undiscovered potential.

In Chinese medicine, *internal organs* refers to much more than the organs themselves. It also refers to a quality of energy described in the Five Elements. The Five Elements are known as the five phases of cyclical energetic movement in both nature and ourselves. For example, the heart is associated with the fire element. The quality of the fire element is expansive, radiant, bright, and warm. The season of the heart is summer, sharing the same qualities of energy. Each organ is associated with a mental and emotional element as well. So each organ has specific characteristics energetically, physically, emotionally, and spiritually. In the human body, the goal of the Taoist practice is to keep the Five Elements in harmony. When the Five Elements are in harmony, the body, mind, and spirit are in balance.

The health of the internal organs greatly affects our sexual energy. Sexual energy is the essence of the internal organs. The body draws the finest energy, especially from the organs, to produce sperm or eggs. When the sexual energy is out of balance, it is reflected in the internal organs, and when one or more organs are out of balance, the sexual energy will definitely be affected. The internal organs and sexual energy are a reflection of each other; when one system is improved, the other follows. To draw and spiral the energy around the organs, sit on the edge of a chair. Gently inhale while contracting the vagina or penis and draw the energy up the spine around the Microcosmic Orbit and out to the organs as the energy comes down the front of your body, directly up from the sexual organs to the five yin and five yang organs in the torso.

The best way to keep the Five Elements in balance and harmony is through the Six Healing Sounds and the Inner Smile. These techniques are discussed in my book *Taoist Ways to Transform Stress into Vitality*. I highly recommend using these techniques to strengthen the energetic quality of the internal organs.

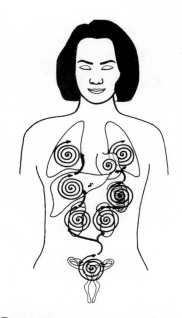

DRAW AND SPIRAL THE ENERGY AROUND THE ORGANS

KIDNEYS AND THE WATER ELEMENT

In Taoist medicine, the kidneys, one of the Five Vital Organs, are a main source of energy. When they are full of energy, one will be energetic and high-spirited, with plenty of stamina and an abundance of sexual energy. This is all because the health of the kidneys is directly related to the health of their corresponding organs, the genitals, and consequently to one's sexual functioning and capability. The kidneys are connected by the Taoists to the ears, thereby making the ears the outlets of the kidneys. By observing the shape and condition of a person's ears, you can determine the general strength and condition of the kidneys.

The kidneys in Chinese medicine represent the water element in the body. Water is associated with the virtue of gentleness and the negative emotion of fear. Gentleness elicits the yin energy of the body. For women, sexual energy is like water. Gentleness stimulates the feminine sexual energy, heating the water element, preparing the body for sexual intercourse.

Female Kidney Energy

To further illustrate the importance of kidney energy as it applies to sexual energy, consider the information set forth in the book entitled *Nei Ching*, the Yellow Emperor's classic text on internal medicine.

The kidney energy of a girl becomes abundant at seven years of age. Her baby teeth begin to be replaced by permanent ones, and her hair begins to grow longer. Her governing meridian is open. At approximately fourteen years of age, a woman begins to menstruate and her conception meridian opens and begins to flow, increasing the energy of her connective meridians in great profusion. With menstruation (called in the classics "Sea of Blood," the Chung Mai) the uterus is now complete and she is capable of impregnation. At the age of twenty-one, the kidney energy of a woman becomes full. As she reaches adulthood, all her teeth are fully developed and her last molars are in. Her "Yang Ming" meridians are now full and connect to her face. She is most radiant and beautiful at this time.

This description serves as one example of how the development of the internal organs can be understood from the manifestation of external factors (for example, teeth, hair, and menstruation), all of which combined indicate the level of the kidneys' development.

Therefore, all the surface structures of the body (the eyes, ears, teeth, nose, fingers, and so on) are relevant to human sexuality because they reflect the internal organs.

Kidney Massage

Stimulating and energizing the kidneys is vitally important to healthy sexual energy. Place both hands over the kidneys, on the low back directly above the last rib. Begin to massage the kidney area vigorously with the palms, feeling the heat penetrate deep into the kidneys. Rub vigorously from the lower back, over the kidneys, and down to the sacrum. Feel this entire area open and energize. After a few minutes of massaging, rest the palms over the

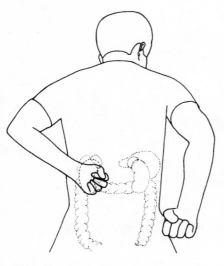

GENTLY HITTING THE KIDNEYS WILL HELP TO SHAKE OUT SEDIMENT

kidneys and project energy into the kidneys. You can visualize a bright blue light penetrating into the kidneys, transforming any negative energy into positive.

Another very beneficial way to stimulate the kidneys is by gently knocking or tapping the lower back area lightly with a loose fist. Knock all the way down to the sacrum and back up to the kidneys, bringing this vibration into the entire lower back area. Do this about nine times.

Massage the Ears

The ears, according to Chinese medicine, are an extension of the kidney energy. One way to stimulate more energy in the kidneys is to massage the ears. The ears have over 120 pressure points. This directly activates sexual energy. That is why couples naturally kiss, nibble, and caress each other's ears.

Place the ear between the thumb and the first finger. Massage the whole ear, giving ample pressure to stimulate energy into the entire body. Kissing or nibbling gently on your partner's ears is a way to activate and bring sexual energy through the whole body.

HEART AND THE FIRE ELEMENT

The heart has a strong connection to the sexual center. It is associated with the fire element and is the energetic center of passion and affection. It is known as the "king" of all the internal organs, circulating blood and energy through the entire system. The fire element is associated with the virtues of love and joy and with the negative emotions of hatred and cruelty. Negative emotions are elicited when energy is not flowing or when energy is congested in the heart. Have you ever noticed that when you do not communicate what is in your heart and instead hold in your emotions, there is a feeling of congestion? This is how negative energy is formed. Energy becomes negative when it is not flowing. Energy stuck in the heart is one of the biggest sexual problems we face. When the energy in the heart is blocked, it is difficult to feel deeply and connect with your partner. For example, when someone in a relationship does not communicate what is in his or her

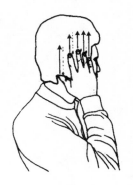

Rub in front and back of ears

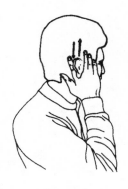

Rub the ear shells

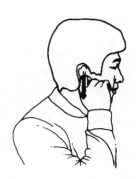

Pull down on the earlobes

CHI EAR SELF-MASSAGE

heart, energy is congested and negative emotions ensue. Expressing what is in our heart in a clear, controlled manner frees this energy and transforms it into something positive.

It is very healthy to establish the intimate connection between the heart and the sexual center. The Tao regards loving energy and sexual energy as the two strongest energies in the body.

Fire energy is also associated with excitement and exhilaration. It is the fire energy in the heart that opens the sexual center. This is why falling in love leads to sexual desire. Many of the Taoist meditations focus on balancing the heart and the sexual center. Even the higher-level Taoist meditations, called Kan and Li (Fire and Water), work on unifying these two energies and steaming their potent force through all the meridians.

Tongue Kung Fu

The tongue is the sense organ of the fire element and the energetic extension of the heart. Exercising the tongue is a great way to open the heart and activate the sexual energy.

There is a very strong connection between the tongue, heart, and sexual center. This is why lovers kiss with the tongue. In some cultures kissing with the tongue is just as intimate as making love.

To exercise the tongue, bring the tip of the tongue in front of the upper teeth inside the lips. Circle the tongue down to the inside lower lip. Continue to circle in front of the teeth and inside the lips about thirty-six times and then switch directions.

Next, massage the flat top part of the tongue by sliding it against the upper palate vigorously. Feel the heat that is generated through the head and the whole body. Heat is a good sign that the fire element is activated in the heart and sexual center. Massage the tongue against the upper palate at least thirty-six times.

Massage the Chest to Open the Heart

Massage the chest with the fingers or knuckles. The knuckles are good to use for deeper pressure. Look for tender areas along the sternum and between the ribs along the chest. Press into them gently, massaging until you feel a release. It is especially good to spend time massaging the sternum, releasing emotional energy

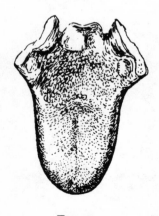

TONGUE

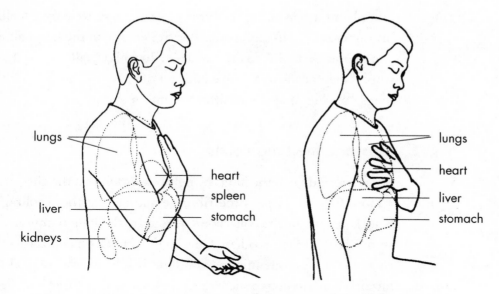

PLACE THE PALM ON THE CHEST TO OPEN THE HEART

that has congested in the heart center. To end, place the hands over the chest and project energy into the heart area. Visualize a bright red, warm glow in the heart. Feel the connection between the heart and the sexual center.

LUNGS AND THE METAL ELEMENT

The lungs are the organs of breath, keeping us intimately connected to the universe. When inhaling, we take in the body of the universe and when exhaling we give back part of ourselves to the universe. The breath is a metaphor of this dynamic exchange of energy. It represents giving and receiving, ebb and flow, male and female. Simply by observing the dynamics of the breath, we can witness the balance of yin and yang and the constant flow and exchange of life-force energy within the universe. Male and female relationships are part of this universal exchange, creating harmony and balance in all apparent opposites.

The breathing patterns always reflect how we feel. When we become sexually aroused, the breath becomes deep and full, pumping energy through the whole body. If the lung energy is weak or congested, it is difficult to feel aroused and excited. The negative energy of the lungs is depression. Depression is one of the biggest causes of impotence and low sexual energy. On the other hand, when energy is flowing in the lungs, we have a feeling of courage and self-expression. Positive energy in the lungs allows you to breathe in life, to experience it. To feel sexually aroused, the whole body needs to be alive and full of energy. This is what the lungs do when they are healthy and full of energy.

Massage the Lung Points

Stimulate and open the lungs by lightly knocking on the chest with a loose fist. This opens the rib cage and relaxes the diaphragm. Knock just below the collarbone to activate the lung points and to stimulate the lung meridian. Continue to knock on and across the chest for at least one minute with both hands. Afterward, feel the buzzing and tingling in the chest area. Take two or three long deep breaths. Feel the lungs open and energize.

LIVER AND THE WOOD ELEMENT

The liver is associated with the wood element and the virtues of kindness and forgiveness. The negative emotions of the liver are frustration (sexual frustration) and anger. When the liver energy is congested, we simply cannot relax. Relaxation is an indispensable quality of good sexual health. When we are tense and tight, energy does not flow.

The liver transfers a tremendous amount of energy to the sexual center. The wood element plays a vital role in the strength of the erection for men and provides the expansive energy for the swelling of the vagina when the woman is sexually aroused. When the wood energy is blocked, men usually have a difficult time getting an erection, even though they may feel aroused. Women may have a difficult time feeling orgasmic. Deep relaxation usually solves these problems. Releasing the congestion in the liver allows the wood energy to flow into the sexual center.

Massage the Feet

The liver meridian runs down the legs and into the feet. Massaging the feet is a great way to relax the body and stimulate the wood element. Whenever the body is able to relax deeper, the sexual center benefits. When the body is under stress and tight, the sexual energy is constricted. Massage the feet with both hands. Pay particular attention to the big toe. This is where the liver meridian ends. Spend at least five minutes on each foot to ensure that the energy moves into the body. If you want to boost your partner's sexual energy immediately, suck or nibble on the big toe.

SPLEEN AND THE EARTH ELEMENT

The spleen is associated with the earth element and the virtues of balance and openness. The negative emotions associated with the spleen are worry and anxiety. When the earth element is out of balance, the feelings of the body are disconnected, making it difficult to get in touch with sensation. For example, when the energy of the spleen is congested, it causes the mind to be overactive. The overactivity in the mind is what causes worry and anxiety. When there is excess energy in the head, it is hard to be in touch with the body.

When energy is flowing in the earth element, we are able to feel our center and our connections to all life. When we feel connected to ourselves, we are able to connect to others, both sexually and emotionally.

Massage the Abdomen

Massage the abdomen in a gentle circle, rubbing with the flow of digestion, from left to right. The abdomen is the center of the body. When the abdomen is full of energy, the body is full of energy. (To understand more about the internal organs and the energy of the abdomen, it is advisable to read my book *Internal Organ Massage*.) Continue to circle the hands around the abdomen at least thirty-six times. With the fingertips, feel for any tightness or congestion. Work into the abdomen and feel the release of tightness. Work with your breathing while you are massaging. See if you can breathe all the way into the belly. Remember, the organs provide energy to the sexual center. When the energy in the abdominal area is full, the sexual center is balanced and harmonized.

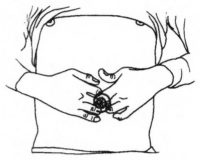

The major key to maintaining good health is to eliminate tension, worry, and toxins every day and maintain good sexual energy by massaging the abdomen.

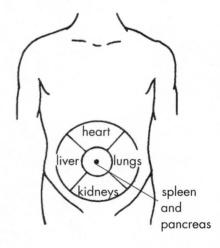

MASSAGING THE ABDOMEN

Secret Art of the Jade Chamber

In *The Classic of the Arcane Maid*, an ancient Taoist text, the Elemental Maid discloses the Art of the Bedchamber to the Yellow Emperor. The positions and secrets she shared will bring great health and pleasure.

There is no joy in yang without yin, and yin without yang is unexcited. In such cases, the man desires copulation but the woman is unhappy, or the woman desires copulation but the man lacks desire. When hearts are out of tune, there is no arousal of the essences. Thus love and pleasure are not forthcoming. However, if the man courts the woman and the woman the man, there is a merging of both minds and desires. They take delight in each other's hearts. Upon the arousal of the woman's passions, she fondles the man's jade stalk and provides it with the power necessary to tap her jewel terrace. This brings an abundance of secretions from both. The jade stalk, greatly enlarged, moves sometimes slowly, sometimes quickly. The jade gate opens to ease the entrance of the powerful adversary and absorb its essence, which irrigates the scarlet chamber.

In responding to the man's yang, the woman shows the following symptoms: Her ears are hot as though she had drunk rich wines. Her breasts protrude firmly so that they fill his hands. The neck moves and the legs shake in an agitated fashion. She attempts to hold back her lascivious movements, but all at once she clings to his body and presses hers deeply against him and gently palpates it. (This describes a basic technique in Chinese massage, which aims at accupoints. The erotic variety of such acupressure acts as a very effective aphrodisiac.)

Next the text goes on to explain to the emperor the reason for awaiting the Four Attainments. It says that "if the jade stalk is not angry, the man's harmonious essence has not yet arrived. If it is stiff but not hot, his spirit muscle essence has not arrived. If it is big but not yet stiff, the bone essence has not yet arrived. Should it be rigid but not hot, the spirit essence has not arrived." In order to perform, all four conditions must be met—even if the man already has an erection.

Next the emperor inquires about a woman's Nine Essences. He wonders what they are and how he can tell whether they have been aroused. The Arcane Maid says, "When a woman deeply sighs and swallows, the essence of her lungs has been aroused. If she utters little cries and sucks his mouth, the heart essence has been aroused. When her yin gate is damp and slippery, the kidney essence has been aroused. Should she enfold and hold him, her spleen essence has been aroused. When she gently bites him, her bone essence has been aroused. Finally, when she caresses his jade stalk, the essence of her blood is aroused."

The Elemental Maid outlines the Five Desires: "If a woman bates her breath and restrains her energy, her mind desires sexual union. If both her nostrils and mouth are dilated, her vulva wants union. If she suddenly embraces the man, she wants to climax. If her perspiration drenches her clothes, she wants her heart filled. If she straightens her body and closes her eyes, she is near ecstasy."

Next the Five Symptoms in the woman are mentioned and a recommendation for the appropriate male response is given. "When her face is flushed, gradually start intercourse. When her breasts are full and her nose perspires, slowly put in the jade stalk. When her throat is dry and she is swallowing, unhurriedly rock the jade stalk. When her grotto is slippery, slowly penetrate to her depths. When her fluids flow to her buttocks, slowly remove the jade stalk." Although the Elemental Maid appears to be giving advice to the male, her instructions are only for the early stages of the encounter, before it becomes more passionate.

In addition, the Elemental Maid discusses the Ten Movements

of a woman in the sweet agony of passion and urges her to be strong: "If she holds him with her arms, she desires to press their bodies together and for their genitals to touch. Should she extend her thighs, she wants to rub her upper vulva against him. If she holds in her stomach, she wants to have an orgasm. If she shakes her buttocks, she desires to be sliced deeply to the left and right. If she lifts up her body against his, her libidinous joy is great. If she stretches out lengthwise, her limbs and body are pleased. If her sexual fluids are slippery, she has attained orgasm. Look at these movements in the 'Original Nine Postures' and you will know how avid is her ecstasy."

ARCANE MAID'S ORIGINAL NINE POSTURES

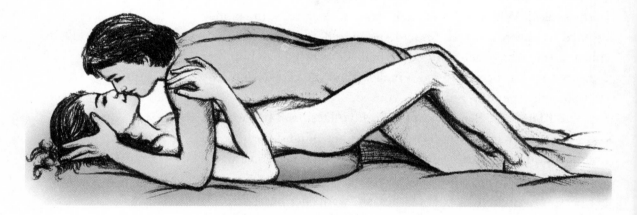

SOMERSAULTING DRAGONS

Somersaulting Dragons ◆ The woman reclines on her back with the man prostrate over her. She presses her thighs into the bed. Taking his jade stalk, she pulls at her vulva. He drives at her grain seed and assails her upper part with leisurely, calculated stokes—eight shallow and two deep. Going in dead, the stalk returns alive, so that he becomes vigorous and strong. She is agitated yet pleased, joyous like a singing maiden. To refrain from ejaculation disperses a hundred illnesses.

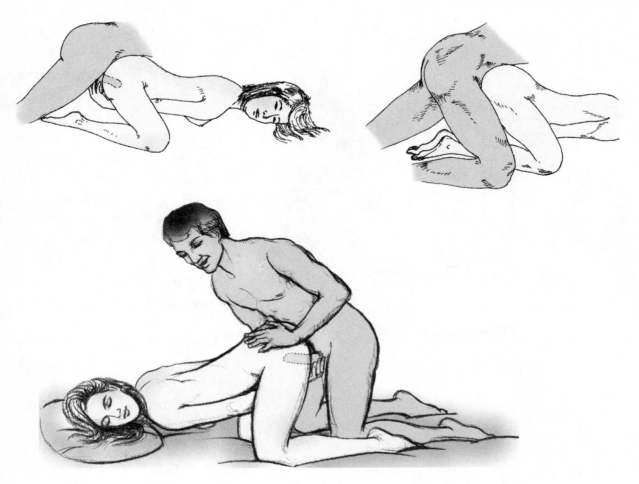

STEPPING TIGERS

Stepping Tigers ◆ The woman takes a crawling position, with the buttocks upward while the head is down. Kneeling behind her, the man clasps her stomach. He inserts his jade stalk, piercing the innermost part of her as deeply and intimately as possible. They take turns advancing and attacking, eight thrusts, five times. As her fluids seep out of her, the jade gate closes and opens. A rest is taken after this occurs. The man will become more virile and a hundred sicknesses will disappear. The Arcane Maid terms this Stepping Tigers, since the participants advance and retreat like a pair of tigers. In such a position the jade stalk refrains from stimulating the clitoris but may penetrate to the flower heart. "Eight thrusts, five times" denotes a total of forty thrusts, with a brief pause after each set of eight.

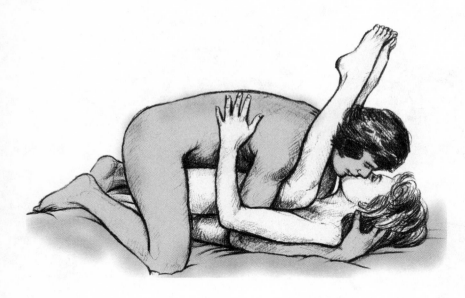

WRESTLING APES

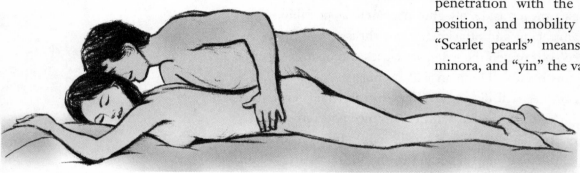

CLEAVING CICADAS

Wrestling Apes ◈ The woman lies on her back, with her knees bent toward her head, and the man supports her thighs, pushes her knees beyond her breasts, raising her buttocks and back. He inserts his jade stalk and stabs her scented mouse. She shakes and rocks. Her fluids flow like rain. He pushes in deeply, without moving. The jade stalk grows strong and angry. He stops when she exults. One hundred sicknesses cure themselves.

Cleaving Cicadas ◈ The woman lies on her stomach and extends her body. Lying on her back, the man inserts his jade stalk deeply. He lifts up her bottom slightly so that he can gently tap her scarlet pearls for a total of nine thrusts, six times. Excited, her fluids flow. Her inside yin throbs quickly, while the outside spreads and opens. He stops when she rejoices. Seven injuries eliminate themselves. (There is fairly shallow penetration with the rear-entry position, and mobility is limited. "Scarlet pearls" means the labia minora, and "yin" the vagina.)

Mounting Tortoises ◈ The woman lies on her back with her knees bent. The man presses her feet until the knees are at her breasts. He puts in his jade stalk deeply and at times stabs at her infant girl. Carefully thrusting deep and shallow, he reaches her grain seed. She is overcome by great joy, shakes, and then lifts her torso. At the point when her fluids overflow, he pierces more deeply and then stops when she rejoices. If no semen is lost, his vigor will multiply a hundredfold. (In this position, which is similar to Wrestling Apes, the man holds the woman's legs instead of her buttocks. It was another favorite ancient Chinese position allowing deep penetration and high mobility. "Infant girl" means the vestibular glands between the labia minora.)

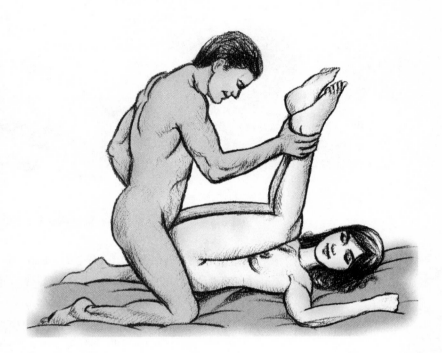

MOUNTING TORTOISES

Soaring Phoenix ◈ The woman lies down and raises her legs while the man kneels between her thighs. His hands are on the bed. He slips his jade stalk in deeply and it pierces her mixed rock. He guides it in, rigid and hot, and requests that she start moving. There are eight thrusts, three times. As their buttocks swiftly attack one another, her yin opens and expands, gushing out its fluids. He halts upon her rejoicing and a hundred illnesses will vanish. (Coital movements here are done mostly by the woman. The "phoenix" refers to the Chinese mythical *feng huang* bird. "Mixed rock" means four inches deep.)

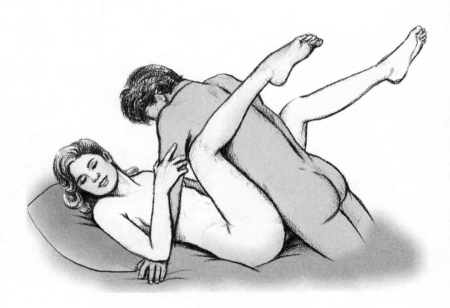

SOARING PHOENIX

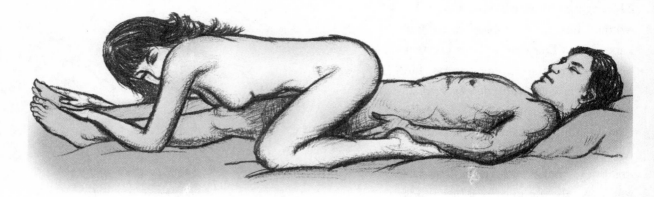

BUNNY LICKING ITS FUR

Bunny Licking Its Fur ◆ The man stretches his legs straight as he lies on his back. The woman straddles his body with her knees to his sides. She faces his feet with her back to his head, holding on to the bed. As she lowers her head, his jade stalk is inserted until it pierces her lute strings. She celebrates as her fluids gush like a fountain. She is delighted with harmonious pleasure, which moves her spirit and body. Upon her rejoicing he halts. A hundred illnesses will not come about. ("Lute strings" symbolizes one inch inside the vagina. With such shallow penetration, the woman needs some practice to forestall the dislocation of their organs. "Licking bunny" means the male organ.)

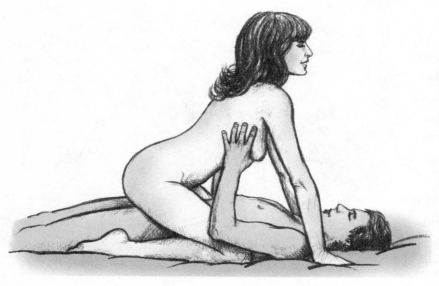

Fish Linking Scales ◆ The man lies flat on his back with the woman over him straddling his body. She carefully and slowly inserts his jade stalk, stopping when he is only a little way in. He does not penetrate deeply, and he imitates a baby sucking at the breast. The woman rocks as he sucks her breasts for a long period. He removes his stalk when she rejoices. This cures all clogging sicknesses.

FISH LINKING SCALES

Cranes Entwining Necks ◈
While the man squats, the woman rides his thighs, her hands holding his neck. She inserts him, letting his jade stalk cut through her wheat bud and jab her seed. He clasps her bottom to help her rocking and rising motions. Feeling wonderful joy, her fluids flow and bubble. He halts when she rejoices. The seven injuries will be healed naturally. (This is another position with the woman above, so it gives her a bit less mobility and shallower penetration. "Wheat bud" is two inches deep, and "seed" means her clitoris.)

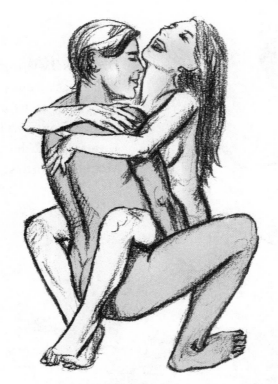

CRANES ENTWINING NECKS

MYSTICAL THIRTY POSTURES

The Mystic Master saw his thirty positions as an amplification of the Arcane Maid's original nine positions. Naming each position, he offers a very short, and sometimes cryptic, description. His positions are simply illustrations, with no trace of motion. However, immediately after the positions, he puts forth the dynamic parts of sexual intercourse.

Entangled Silkworms ◈ Lying on her back, the woman hugs the man's neck with her feet crossed above his back. He puts his knees between her spread thighs while grasping her neck. Then he inserts his jade stalk.

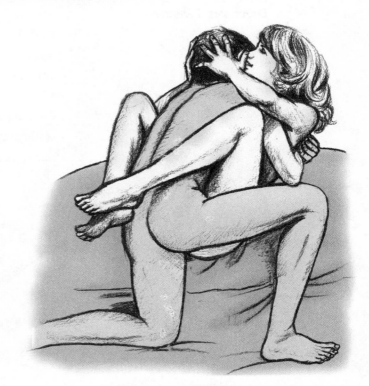

ENTANGLED SILKWORMS

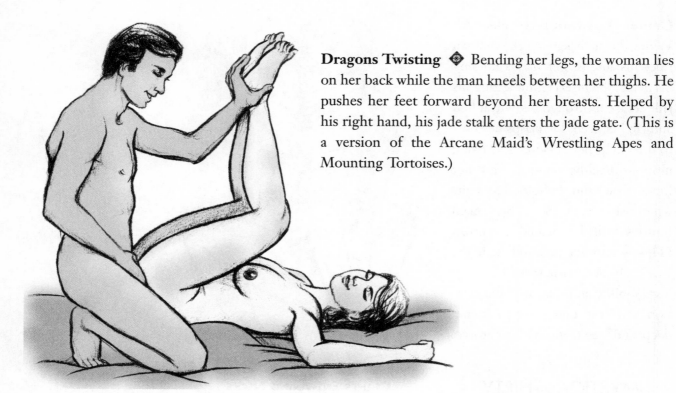

Dragons Twisting ◈ Bending her legs, the woman lies on her back while the man kneels between her thighs. He pushes her feet forward beyond her breasts. Helped by his right hand, his jade stalk enters the jade gate. (This is a version of the Arcane Maid's Wrestling Apes and Mounting Tortoises.)

DRAGONS TWISTING

Fish Eye to Eye ◈ This position calls for the couple to lie down facing each other. They proceed to suck one another's lips and tongues. The woman raises one leg above the man's body and he spreads his legs slightly. One hand supports her upraised leg. He slips his jade stalk into her cinnabar grotto. (This position frees the partners from bearing each other's body weight.)

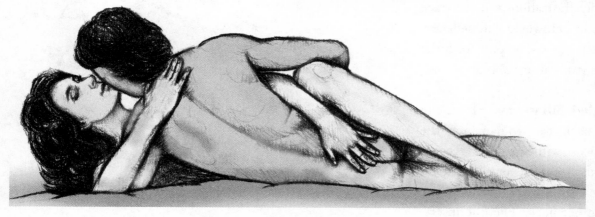

FISH EYE TO EYE

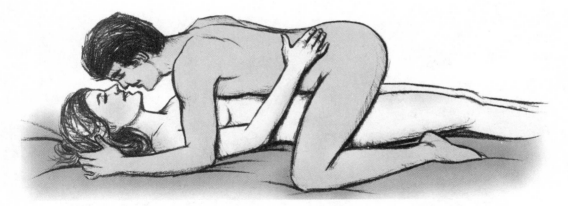

SWIFTS SHARING A HEART

Swifts Sharing a Heart ◈ The woman reclines on her back and stretches out her legs. The man squats over her stomach while his hands embrace her neck. She holds his waist with her hands. He slides his jade stalk into her cinnabar grotto.

Kingfishers Uniting ◈ The woman reclines on her back, knees raised. The man puts himself between her thighs in a Tartar squat. (The Tartar squat is a traditional position of people from northern China.) He holds her waist with his hands and puts his jade stalk into her lute strings (one inch into the vagina).

KINGFISHERS UNITING

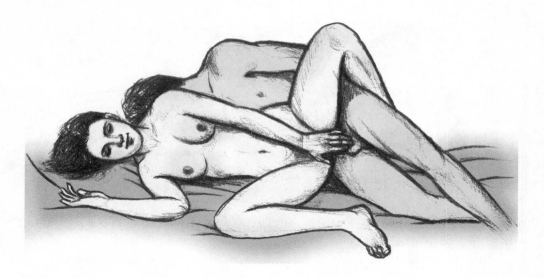

MANDARIN DUCKS JOINING

Mandarin Ducks Joining ◈ The woman bends her legs while reclining on her side. The man reclines behind her, facing her back. She places her upper leg on the man's buttocks. He rides on her lower thigh, lifting one knee up against her upper thigh. He then slides in his jade stalk.

BUTTERFLIES FLUTTERING

Butterflies Fluttering ◈ While the man reclines on his back with his legs extended, the woman sits astride him facing his head. With her feet on the bed, she uses her hand to put his yang peak into her jade gate.

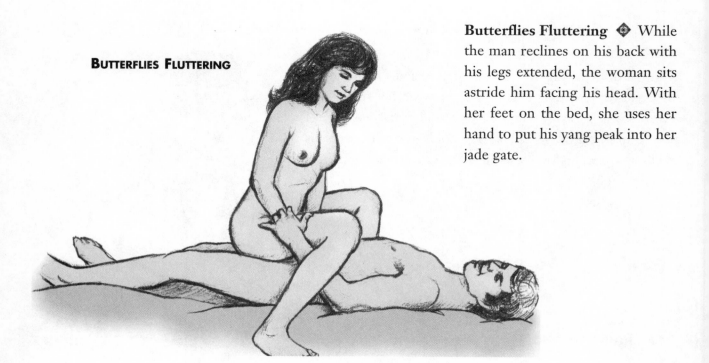

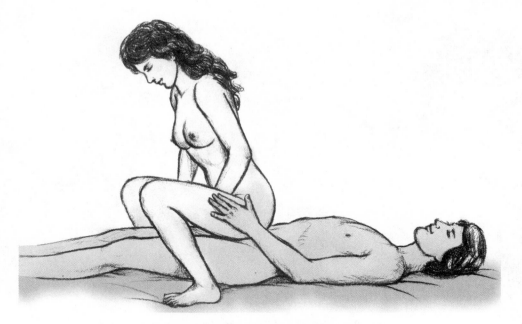

WILD DUCKS FLYING BACKWARD

Wild Ducks Flying Backward ❖ The man reclines on his back and stretches out his legs. The woman sits down on him with her face toward his feet and uses her feet to support herself on the bed. She lowers her head, takes his jade stalk, and inserts it into the cinnabar grotto.

Sheltering the Reclining Pine ❖ The woman reclines on her back and folds her feet behind the man's waist. They hold each other's waists as he inserts his jade stalk into her jade gate.

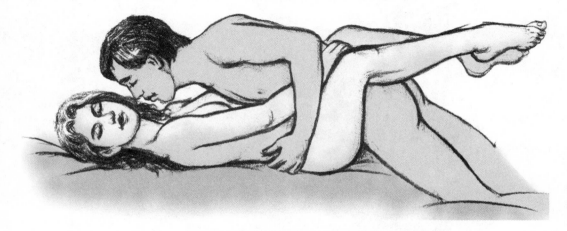

SHELTERING THE RECLINING PINE

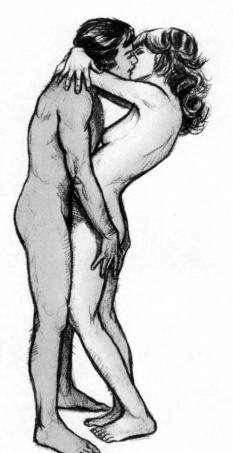

BAMBOO BY THE ALTAR

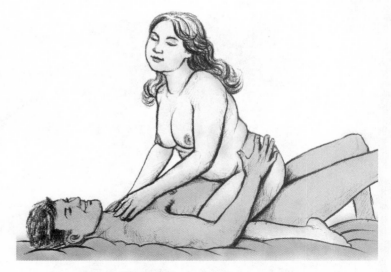

PHOENIX HOLDING FLEDGLINGS

Bamboo by the Altar ◈ Here, the man and woman stand, facing each other, and embrace and kiss. He slices her cinnabar grotto deeply with his yang peak, all the way down to her yang terrace.

Phoenix Holding Fledglings ◈ A large heavy woman can be joined by a smaller man to make a good love union. This is fine excellence!

Seagulls Soaring ◈ The man stands near the edge of the bed, where he lifts the woman's legs high and inserts his jade stalk deeply into her baby palace.

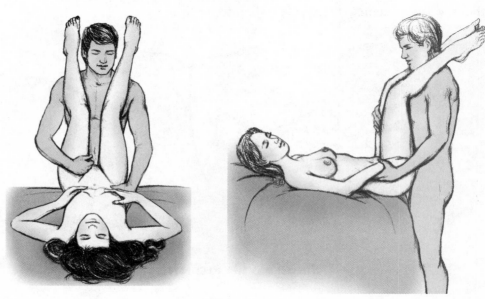

SEAGULLS SOARING

Wild Horses Leaping ◈ The man lifts the woman's feet while she is on her back and puts them on his shoulders. He slides the jade stalk deep into the jade gate.

Steeds Galloping ◈ The woman reclines on her back. The man extends his body over hers and holds her neck with one hand while the other hand lifts her leg. He puts his jade stalk into her baby palace.

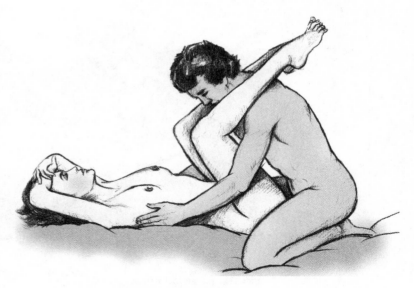

WILD HORSES LEAPING

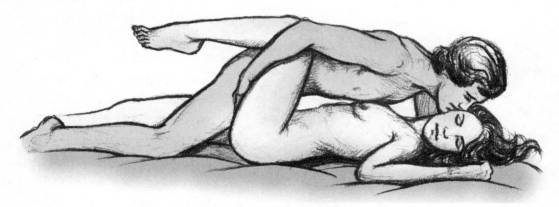

STEEDS GALLOPING

HORSE SHAKING ITS HOOF

Horse Shaking Its Hoof ◈ The man puts one of the woman's legs on his shoulder while she lifts the other one herself. The man puts his jade stalk deep into the cinnabar grotto. This is very arousing.

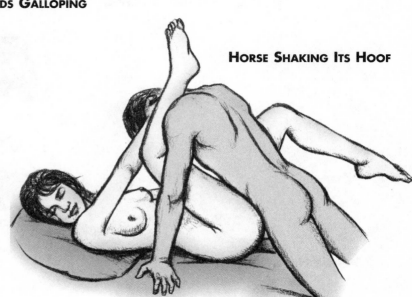

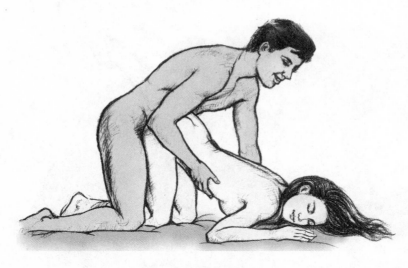

WHITE TIGER JUMPING

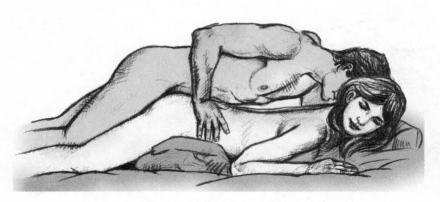

DUSKY CICADAS CLEAVING

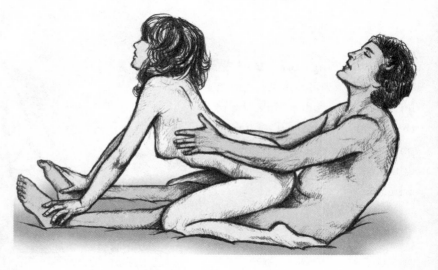

GOAT HUGGING THE TREE

White Tiger Jumping ✦ The woman kneels and her face is lowered. The man, hands holding her waist, kneels behind her and inserts his jade stalk into her baby palace.

Dusky Cicadas Cleaving ✦ The woman lies on her stomach and extends her legs. With his legs bent between her thighs, the man holds her neck with his hand. He then inserts his jade stalk into the jade gate from behind.

Goat Hugging the Tree ✦ The man is seated with legs extended. With her back to his face, the woman sits on his lap. As she lowers her head to look at the insertion of his jade stalk, he abruptly holds her waist, bridling and thrusting.

Jungle Fowl Approaching the Arena ◈ The man crouches Tartar style on the bed as a young maidservant grasps his jade stalk. She proceeds to insert it into the jade gate of his partner. The maid then stands back and tugs the hems of the other woman's skirt to stimulate her legs. Very rousing!

Phoenix Sporting in the Cinnabar Grotto ◈ The woman lifts her feet as she reclines on her back. The man rests on his knees at her buttocks holding on to the bed. He enters into her cinnabar grotto with his jade stalk. Extremely courtly!

Rock Soaring over Dark Sea ◈ As the woman lies on her back, the man puts her feet on his upper arms. Stretching his hands down to hold her waist, he puts in his jade stalk.

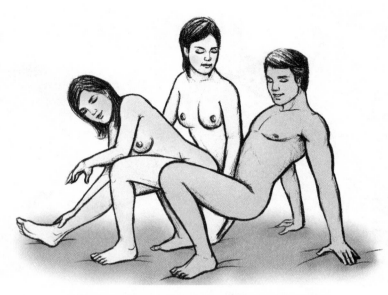

JUNGLE FOWL APPROACHING THE ARENA

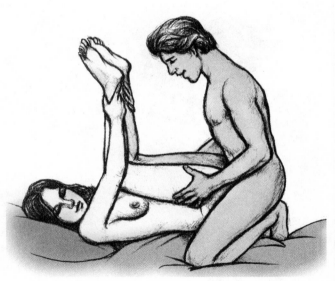

PHOENIX SPORTING IN THE CINNABAR GROTTO

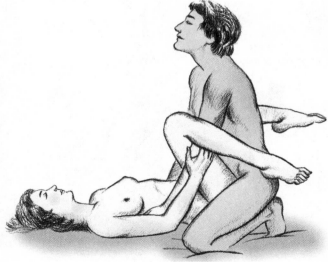

ROCK SOARING OVER DARK SEA

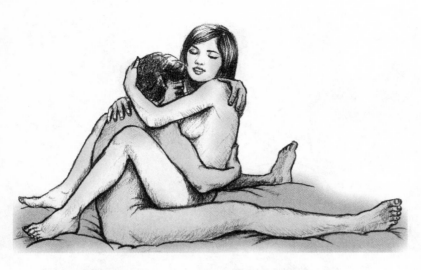

HUMMING APE EMBRACING THE TREE

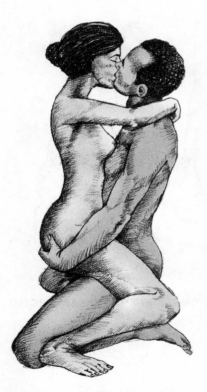

**CAT AND MOUSE SHARING
A HOLE**

Humming Ape Embracing the Tree ◆ While seated, the man stretches out his legs. The woman spans his thighs and holds him. One of his hands holds her buttocks, and the other holds the bed. He slips in his jade stalk.

Cat and Mouse Sharing a Hole ◆ The man kneels upright on his knees. The woman squats on top of him, thighs apart, and his jade stalk is penetrating deep inside her.

Donkeys of Spring ◆ The woman grasps the bed with both her hands and feet. The man embraces her waist from behind with his hands. He slips the jade stalk into her jade gate. Quite stately!

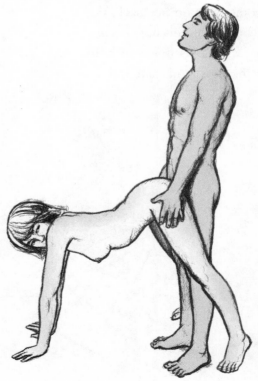

DONKEYS OF SPRING

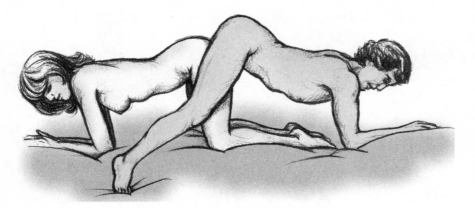

DOG OF AUTUMN

Dog of Autumn ◈ Both the man and the woman grip the bed with their hands and feet. They are back to back, haunches pressed together. The man lowers his head and uses his hand to push his jade stalk into the jade gate.

Spider Trapped in Its Own Hole ◈ Here the woman hangs free from a set of ropes attached to the ceiling. It is similar to a swing or riding on a horizontal bar. Her thighs are spread. The man inserts his jade flute into her cinnabar field. The maid assists with positioning the woman above the man.

Feast of Ponies ◈ The man lies on his back. One woman rides him and another sits on his face. (It should be mentioned that in ancient China, this was a perfectly respectable family union in a country that was traditionally polygamous.)

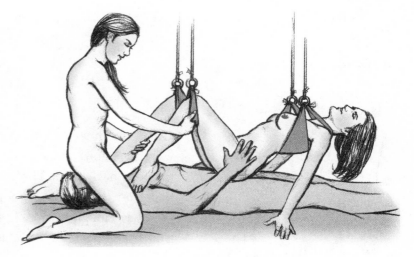

SPIDER TRAPPED IN ITS OWN WEB

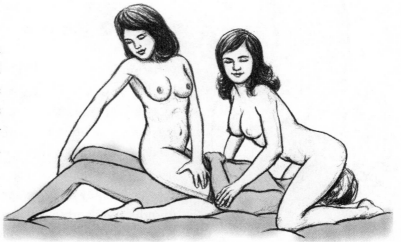

FEAST OF PONIES

OLD MAN PUSHING THE WHEELBARROW

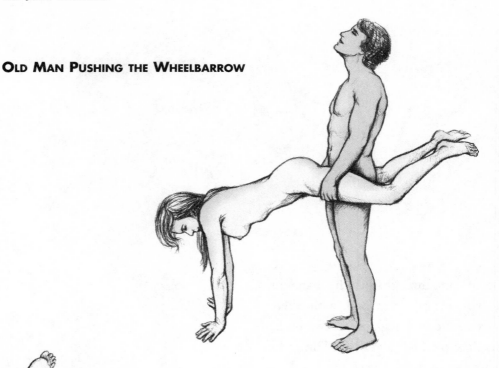

Old Man Pushing the Wheelbarrow ✦ This position is some-what strenuous. It usually begins with the woman on all fours near the edge of the bed. The man stands behind her and inserts his jade stalk from the rear. The woman stretches her legs. The man holds her thighs as though he were holding the handles of a wheelbarrow. Her hands support her and she faces the floor. They stay attached as he moves backward away from the bed, while she walks her hands down from the bed. She walks on her hands, coordinating her movement with his. The man walks her forward around the room.

Scissors ✦ This position has both a horizontal and a vertical version. They feature a different angle of insertion. The horizontal variation is very restful. The woman reclines on her side and raises her upper thigh. The man lies on his back with his head near her feet and spreads his thighs. He moves in between her thighs. Their legs move like two pairs of scissors trying to cut each other. The vertical variation is much more strenuous. The woman stands on her head, her body and legs raised upward with the help of the man. He stands between her spread thighs. The woman holds up her upright body with her hands as the man pierces her by bending his knees and moving up and down.

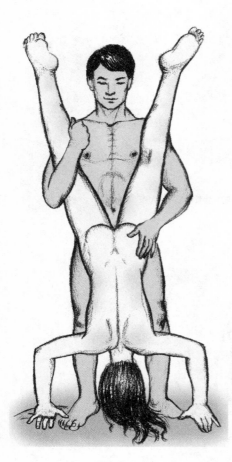

SCISSORS

12

Romancing the Moon Grotto

This commentary is taken from *Yin-Yang Butterfly* by Valentin Chu and gives you the idea and feeling of romancing the moon grotto (vagina) with the Pluck and Nurture techniques from the Art of the Bedchamber practiced in fourteenth-century China.

Similar to a riffling dragon, the pale wall with its wavelike, tiled top encloses the hidden garden. On the distant side, bamboo swings in the energizing breezes of a summer's day. Goldfish swim lazily in an irregularly fashioned pool framed with greenery and bridged by a slim, arched span of bright cinnabar. To one side a low, meandering house with curled eaves and upswept roof corners can be found. The scent from a bunch of jasmine bushes provides an uplifting sensuousness to the breeze.

Sipping warm rice wine from dainty ceramic cups and nibbling delicacies from several plates, a man and woman sit by a table near a huge boulder. The maidservant who served the dishes has quickly left. The man and woman talk in quiet voices. As he continues to talk, a long, loose sleeve of his muslin robe hits a pair of chopsticks and they fall off the table. He bends over, squatting under the table to pick them up. Instead his hand touches the woman's petite, delicate foot.

"Oh!" the woman exclaims, seemingly alarmed. The man starts fondling her feet. She blushes a lurid pink. Standing up,

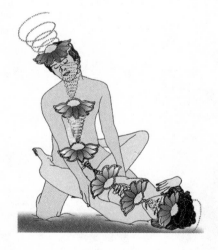

PLUCK AND NURTURE TECHNIQUE

the man walks to her side. He holds her cringing shoulders with his hands and places his nose next to the back side of her neck to give a sniff-kiss. "Oh, please stop!" she whispers in protest. As his sniff-kisses slowly move to her cheek, she abruptly turns her face and gives him a full kiss on the mouth. She always has appeared coy and acted like a woman of good breeding. Now he knows better. Such women are all alike, with their frigid attitudes but hot lips, modest glances but hard nipples. Often he has noticed a secret curvaceousness in this striking young widow, and he has patiently tried to trap her for months. Their mating dance has been lengthy and hidden behind traditional manners and highly indirect coded messages. Their time-consuming signals and interaction finally made her agree to this supper in his stately garden.

The couple strolls into the house, whispering to each other as they go. They go into the bedchamber. The room contains a huge traditional bedstead, which is practically a room unto itself. A precisely carved ebony lattice frame guards three of the bed's sides. Inside the latticework there is a wraparound muslin curtain. The two flaps in front are held up with a pair of big silver hooks. Beads and semi-precious stones hang from them.

Immediately upon sitting on the bed, they start kissing again. He slowly begins taking off her clothes: her waistband, her silk gown, her sleeveless undergarment, her bodice, and finally her underpants. Her partial resistance combined with partial concession only serve to arouse his eagerness. When they are naked, he views the luscious banquet before him. The almond eyes, the red-red mouth and the naked arms remind him of clean-scrubbed lotus roots. Her breasts are like fresh hills of new tofu with a freshly peeled lotus seed on top.

He is now ready to experience her fineness. When he does, he will add to her essence for his purpose. This will be a wonderfully delicious banquet of longevity. He pays respect to every part of her scrumptious body by touching and kissing her. He alternates subtle tenderness with flagrant boldness. Retreating like a fleeing animal, there are occasional stops to flirt and bait him. For an extended period their entire world is a mixture of limbs and loins; of tender warm skin and damp lips.

He takes a moment to look at this awe-inspiring woman. Her transparent, ceramic flesh, damp with sweat, provides a feminine scent. She breathes deeply, quivering slightly with sensuality from her small navel and her slim waist. And then there is her cinnabar palace protruding very slightly with its abundance of being. She takes a recently opened pomegranate with its red pulp and spreads it before him. Now yin and yang are harmonious for a union of exultant happiness.

He starts his hallowed mission into the grotto of love—the mystical grotto—the place where we all enter this world—and the place which grown men strive to enter. As he starts his journey, her black eyes, before half closed in a dreamy velveteen, abruptly open, staring with sharp desire. His skills with the blade have been termed brilliant. His jabs, counters, and returns have conquered the most skilled of bedchamber opponents.

"No! No! No! No!" she gasps to his rhythm.

The silver hooks of the bed drapes clink ever so quietly. The dance of life goes on. While this is an exercise in pleasure for him, it is also of supreme importance. It supercedes ginseng, and is a lot more fun. He rolls her around in different positions. The masters taught him how to elicit the desired effect on her. He recounts without sound to himself the secret words from that astounding volume on sexual alchemy: "The white tiger swings hither and yon. The blue dragon goes upward and downward. The lunar grotto opens and shuts. The celestial root lunges and strums." He thinks: "I must tighten my rectum, hold my breath, and shut all my bodily openings."

Now the dragon grasps the tiger's buttocks and pushes against her bosom. He sucks the tiger's tongue, clutches the midsection, and lifts the knees. "Allow the tiger to move. Let her rock and breathe," he tells himself. The tiger's aureate eyes drift heavenward in elated bliss. "This works fine," he says to himself. The calm chrysanthemum is changing into a dew-covered peony shaking in a helpless manner in the breeze.

After the tiger's golden eyes drift toward the heavens, he can cull her potion. Very soon she will swim in her own love juices. She has to be the most lascivious woman in China. The peony is dripping with dew, but does not give forth its potion. She's delicate, but stronger than he imagined. This struggle might take some time. The best skills of his bed-chamber martial arts must be called into action. He moves on to the ravaging technique of varied thrusts. First he uses nine shallow and one deep thrust. Then he shifts to eight slow and two fast. It seems to be working. The tone of her voice and subtle movements reveal a series of carnal waves in her, yet the mighty burst does not come. She hangs on the edge of the cliff but does not tumble off.

He has to work harder in order to reap her bountiful offerings. Abruptly, there is a piercing warning sound throughout his body. He's on the edge himself. He quickly stops, grasping her to stop her motions. They are two motionless statues. He will start again but first this respite. When they start again he will surely push her over the edge. She is presently absolutely still, yet he senses some tiny palpitations in her moon grotto. Then they grow into spasms. The cinnabar grotto of this wanton female seems to have a life of its own. The grotto opens and closes and squeezes in a most unsettling manner. In seconds, the Yellow River is breaking through its levees. He is ejaculating. His jade stalk, up to now an unvanquishable conqueror, is being exploited helplessly by the throbbing wall of her moon grotto. The flower heart way inside her is eagerly draining his essence.

He is not only defeated but humiliated. He drops to the bed. He feels like an insect sucked dry by a ravenous spider. Devoid of strength, he moans: "What did you do to me! I've had years of cultivation and nurture. Now it is all gone!" She replies softly, "Sir, you are well known for plucking women. You tried mightily for over two hours to draw out my nectar. Instead, you gave me yours." Oblivious to his groaning, she continues. "So is it so wrong for a woman to pluck a man? In the battle of pluck, one must be accepting of defeat as well as triumph." "You have destroyed me," he whines. "You are a wanton fox devil!" "Nonsense! Don't believe in shamans. No man is ruined unless he does it too often. It was pleasurable for both of us and it will keep us both young."

The romancing of the moon grotto love play begins long before a kiss or caress. It might start with a subtle innuendo, a titillating encryption, an audacious sexual invitation. Perhaps the body speaks with a look, a grin, a toss of hair, or a deep breath. Maybe the opening signals begin amid an erotic atmosphere of soft lights, sultry music, the sweet smell of flowers or perfume. Partners well known to each other, especially those married for a long time, often minimize or even skip love play, but occasionally returning to the romantic can refresh and revitalize lovemaking. The physical aspect of love play should be approached carefully. In addition, because intercourse is the most intimate act shared by two people, personal hygiene is of extreme importance.

Men tend to be more genitally oriented than women. Sometimes men might tend to go straight to their partner's genitalia at the beginning of love play. This can reduce the sensitivity of a woman. Quickly beginning sex can be either a potion or a poison—especially for a female. Appropriate do's and don'ts should be respected. As with driving, traffic signs should be followed: "slow," "yield," "stop," "soft shoulder," "curve ahead," "slippery when wet." If one wants to go into uncharted waters, a good plan is to slip in tentatively and slip out immediately. Then observe the partner's reaction. If it is obviously negative, revise your course. If there is halfhearted resistance or ritual, use the Taoist method of two steps forward and one step back. With this tactic in love play, a person can discover unspoken pleasures that both partners secretly want but are loath to speak of directly.

There is no specific time or place for love play. While some lovers, perhaps out of ingenuity or desperation, like the unconventional, or even dangerous, locales, most prefer a romantic environment, perhaps a hidden, moonlit beach or a cozy, dimly lit room, with romantic music or candlelight. It could be the bedchamber, with perhaps the bed strewn with flower petals.

FOREPLAY

The overture to love play can be carefully planned or totally ad lib. A laugh, a glance, a double entendre, a comment from either partner—nearly anything—can touch off a series of wonderful events. When one strokes the partner's palm very slightly with a finger or sucks a fingertip, an all-night conflagration can be ignited. An occasional butterfly kiss here and there on the partner's arm, face, and neck can titillate. Nibbling the earlobe also excites some partners. In fact, some of the accupoints on the ear are love points. The natural aroma of a clean woman can be intoxicating to some men, especially during an erotic moment.

A major element in Chinese erotic poetry is olfactory sensitivity. It is found in the famed poem "Ten Fragrances." In addition, the French use the term *cassolette* (perfume pan) to describe the scent of a woman's body: lips, hair, skin, armpits, vulva, and even her fingertips. This natural womanly odor is best enjoyed with a sniff-kiss, or Chinese kiss. It is done by putting one's nose next to the partner's body and sniffing in a gentle, loving way. The Chinese use this type of kiss as a loving gesture with small children and as a way of flirting. The Chinese reserve lip kissing for an erotic bedroom act.

Sometimes, if a couple is dining in private, it can be stimulating to feed one another. This can vary from spooning food into one another's mouths to transferring food from mouth to mouth. There are numerous foods that are erotic in nature, including peaches, jelly, raw oysters, and clams. Transferring wine from mouth to mouth is an age-old erotic act that tantalizes many couples. There are those who enjoy pouring a little champagne into the bellybutton of their mate and then licking and kissing it. The chilled, fizzing champagne excites some partners. On the other hand, warm rice wine, perhaps Chinese *shaoshing* or Japanese sake, is a good choice too.

A terrific prelude to sex is touch dancing. Many types of dancing evolved from artistic forms and symbolic representations of coitus. Touch dancing permits one to learn a great deal physically about one's partner through rhythm, motion, and bodily interaction even while fully dressed. A discriminating person can intuitively sense the sexual manner of the dance partner. In private, dancing half dressed or naked is an erotic preliminary to love play. Signs of this prelude are frequently high-spirited. Periodic, brief touches done in an apparently accidental way are safe in case of opposition. However, they may be quite arousing to a receptive partner.

There are signals that are particularly effective. This is the case whether dealing with a sexually restrained partner or with a familiar, but until-now platonic, friend. One technique is the "dead hand." Here a person "absentmindedly" and gently places his or her hand on the other's upper arm, shoulder, waist, or thigh. If the person reacts negatively, the hand is quickly removed. However, with no negative reaction, the hand stays without moving, as if dead. If there is a positive reaction, the dead hand becomes increasingly bolder. Another high-spirited gambit is a pinch to some taut, fleshy portion of the body. This could be the shoulder if a person is diffident or the thigh or bottom if one is more venturesome.

The surprise single slap, echoing in the receiver's rear, is an attention-getter at the right moment, for instance when the person is bent over picking something up. Tickling, while usually thought of as being for children, is also fine for grown-ups, because the feeling is decidedly sexual. The most sensitive spots for tickling are the underarms, behind the knees, the bottoms of the feet, the back side of the neck, the sides of the body, and the inner thighs. Friendly wrestling is an infallible prelude to erotic activities. This playful scuffle needs neither a referee nor rules. A handcuff hold by the stronger person might well bring about more interesting activities.

A prelude with excellent physical possibilities is a pillow fight. This bedchamber activity can disperse hidden sexual enmity. Furthermore, it can bring partners to a point of sensual playfulness. It is best to use down pillows that have no buttons, as they make the best weapons. It is possible to hit the other person with gusto and, if done in the right place, not harm him or her in the slightest. There should, however, be no heavy blows to the face, breasts, or genitals. A wild pillow fight might make a mess of feathers, so pillows with synthetic or rag stuffing can be used. The fight can take place while dressed, partially dressed, or completely naked, depending on personal taste and the impulse of the moment.

Undressing oneself quickly shows either great urgency or a lack of diplomacy. Disrobing each other can be a strong source of arousal because it is both enticing and sexually arousing. Undressing can be done slowly, as in a game of strip poker. In this game the loser of each round must take off one or more pieces of clothing.

The mouth, with its soft, pliable tissues and excellent tactile and taste sensors, is an erotic organ. This makes kissing both effective and essential in love play. The mouth is exceedingly open to sensual stimulation. The nerve endings on the lips and tongue are quite sensitive. The mouth itself can react erotically to the touch of a partner's lips, tongue, and, if in the throes of passion, teeth. The amount of suction used determines the sensation. The olfactory cells in the nervous system in the nose are near the mouth. The odor of a partner's breath and mouth and the nearby skin can be highly bracing, especially if it is combined with the quite personal taste of lips and tongue. In erotic mouth-to-mouth kissing, we touch, taste, and smell our partner. This is so intimate that it is akin to coitus. The sensuous kiss can be as soft and changeable as a fluttering butterfly. It may be as deep and lengthy as the famed French kiss practiced by the young people of Pays de Mont in Brittany, where lovers use their tongues to search and explore each other's mouths, sometimes for hours on end. Such penetrating kissing is often the first sexually arousing act between lovers. Very often, depending on the mood and degree of intimacy, it leads to other forms such as caressing.

Not only have modern sexologists outlined the erogenous zones, but Taoists of old mapped assorted love spots on the body. Any part of the body, actually, can be an erogenous zone. Stroking the back of the neck softly, kissing the sides of the neck, probing the ear opening with a tongue, or softly biting the earlobe may arouse a partner a great deal. Other sensuous parts are the underarms or inside the elbows, thighs, and knees. There are erogenous zones at the lower back and, as we all know, in the area of the genitals. The love points mentioned by the ancient Taoists are similar but not identical to the modern erogenous zones. Furthermore, sensitivity in the erogenous zones is different from person to person. Some people have no sensitivity at all in certain areas.

However, some women's breasts are so sensitive that caressing them can bring the woman to orgasm. There are others, though, who are not aroused at all in this fashion. Sensitivity in other areas can vary even more. In general, most people are erotically sensitive in the erogenous zones.

The thoughtful partner first explores and experiments in different areas in love play in order to learn the most effective way to arouse and please the partner. Sensitivity generally increases from the extremities of arms and legs toward the body, and from the outside portions of the torso to the center. Caressing a partner in the peripheral areas and moving to more sensitive areas can create an increase in desire.

Kissing and caressing are a natural combination in love play. In general, a good lover does not go immediately to the genital area or even the breasts. An inexperienced or aggressive lover, frequently the male, is often too bold, direct, and impatient. Such a person roughly grabs the woman's breasts and buttocks, rams his penis in, and ejaculates. This is not only rude and crude but also certain to turn many women off. Gentle and tender caresses, at least at the beginning, are much more likely to arouse a woman. Stronger and more assertive love play is effective when the partner has already become excited. Many men are more aroused by slow and considerate love play as well. Finally, the sight, sound, and odor of an excited mate can frequently be potent aphrodisiacs.

Most women are quite aroused when their breasts are caressed and kissed. There is a significant nerve link between the lips and the breasts, as well as between breasts and genitals. Consequently, mouth-to-mouth kissing can make the nipples become stiff and erect, while stimulating the breasts often makes the clitoris also become erect and the sexual fluids flow.

Starting lovemaking with a good kiss helps ensure a pleasurable experience for both individuals. Some women are a bit more passionate, and more psychological techniques may make their nipples erect. The majority, however, are excited by a combination of psychological and physical factors, including love play at their breasts. After kissing and caressing his partner's face, neck, and shoulders, a good lover moves to her breasts. If done with tenderness and passion, this will greatly stimulate his partner. Most women like having their breasts cupped and lifted with the palms, gently caressed around the nipples, and gently squeezed. They enjoy it when their breasts are kissed and their nipples are rhythmically and playfully licked with the tip of the tongue. Varying erotic sensations can be given to the woman using the smooth (bottom) and rough (top) sides of the tongue alternately. Exciting preliminaries such as this should precede going on to the lower areas of the buttocks, groin, perineum, vulva, and clitoris.

Love play should progress naturally to the area of the genitals. Touching a lover's genitals can be done with the hand, the mouth, or other parts of the body. Next to coitus itself, this is the most passionate and intimate form of sensual communication between lovers. It may be a temporary end in itself, or it may progress to orgasm or intercourse. Caressing the genitals can be done a number of ways, including stroking, fondling, pushing, rubbing, oscillating, tickling, thrusting, kissing, nibbling, licking, and sucking.

These can be done with varying pressure, speed, and rhythm. Some women are enthralled with continuous, persistent caresses, but others prefer a provoking, repeated stop-and-go manner. Since genital organs are made of tender, sensitive tissue, caressing should begin with slow, light touches. After that it can progress to a more active, speedier, heavier approach. This gradual progression allows the participants to be both emotionally and physically prepared. For example, it assists genital lubrication, which prevents discomfort and even pain. Different techniques of caressing are appropriate for different areas of the pubic region. Soft strokes and kisses are most arousing on the insides of both the thighs and the groin. The cinnabar field (the area between the pubic bone and navel) and a woman's mons veneris (pubic bone area) react in a positive manner to a massaging palm. The fleshy buttock can take much heavier caressing, for example, kneading, squeezing, and soft slapping. Stroking the bottom and occasionally moving to the perineum is very provocative. There is a wide range of oral-genital play, including gently kissing the partner's genitals and using the mouth or tongue in a manner similar to intercourse. Some people find this wonderful, while others are disgusted by it.

One of the most sexually sensitive areas, but often overlooked, is the perineum, which is the zone between the anus and the genitals. It corresponds to the *hui-yin* in acupuncture. This area stimulates a male erection in addition to female desire. Caressing the perineum softly with the fingers or the end of the tongue is very energizing.

While many people think of the anus as strictly an organ for excretion, in fact it is connected to sexual nerves, some of which are quite excited when the anus is caressed. Of course it should be thoroughly washed prior to caressing. The French use the word *postillonage* to describe pressing and poking the anus with a finger, and *feuille de rose* (rose leaf) to describe licking it and probing into it with the end of the tongue.

The caressing and the kissing of the genitals necessarily involves genital fluids. These fluids are nature's inventive preparation for intercourse. They lubricate the sexual organs in order to facilitate coitus. In addition, they are a pheromone that acts as a sexual attractant that excites partners. Taoists of old thought that ample lubrication was of supreme importance for enjoyable sex. Modern sexologists, who suggest substitutes such as saliva or artificial lubricants in case of emergency, agree. Natural ingredients, in sex, as with food, are always the best.

Looked at scientifically, genital fluids are similar to saliva. In fact, the genitals, if carefully washed, have fewer bacteria than the mouth. Male genital secretions are a clear, slippery liquid oozing from the opening of the phallus. They come from two pea-size glands just under the prostate as well as several smaller ones in the urethra. Such secretion is not semen, but if the man becomes extremely aroused, there may be a small amount of semen as well. Women have a similar liquid emitted from four vestibular glands around the vaginal opening. When sexually excited, the wall of the vagina also "perspires" a liquid that at times can be quite plentiful. The semen ejaculated by a man during his orgasm originates in the testicles and prostate. It is a gooey, milklike fluid that becomes more liquid when exposed to air. Some experts hold that some women ejaculate a fluid if they have a deep uterine orgasm. This transparent liquid serves no function biologically but is believed to enhance sexual pleasure.

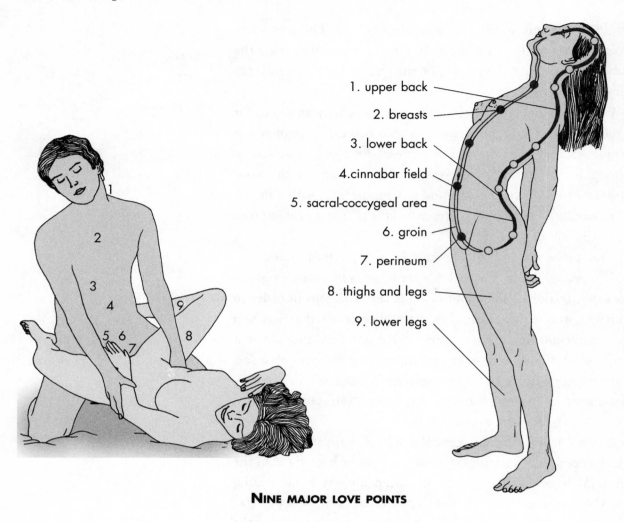

1. upper back
2. breasts
3. lower back
4. cinnabar field
5. sacral-coccygeal area
6. groin
7. perineum
8. thighs and legs
9. lower legs

NINE MAJOR LOVE POINTS

NINE MAJOR LOVE POINTS

Perineum ◈ The sex crossroads is the *hui-yin* and is one of the most important love points. It is located at the middle of the perineum, just barely beneath the skin. Acupuncturists use it in treating penile pain, vaginitis, irregular menstruation, and a prolapsed uterus. In love play, the perineum may be stroked and the point pressed with a fingertip for four seconds, released and pressed again. This is done about forty times, or for five minutes. This spot is one of the two known erection centers for men. (The other one is described below.)

Cinnabar field ◈ There are seven love points in this area from the navel to the pubic symphysis (in front of the pubic bone, felt slightly above the genitals). One way to locate them is to think of the distance from the navel to the pubic symphysis as five sections, each a little over an inch long. The umbilicus itself contains a love point. A segment under it is *yin-chiao* (sexual crossroads). Half a section below is *chi-hai* (sea gate). This is a major love point within the cinnabar field. Half a section below that is *shih-men* (stone gate). Continuing downward, at the bottom of each of the next three sections are *kuen-yuan* (pass of primacy), *chung-chi* (ultimate middle), and *chu-ku*, the pubic bone. All seven of these love points are closely tied to sexual well-being and sexual desire. While participating in love play, each of them should be stroked and pressed with the palm. They should never be pressed heavily with the fingertips but lightly. Press each for three to five seconds and then release and repeat. The downward movement from the navel to the genital region using gentle acupressure at each point increases the partner's arousal. The tongue, if made stiff, can be used instead of a finger.

Breasts ◈ The love points on women's breasts can be used for short-term arousal or long-term engagement. Both nipples have love points. The breastbone, at the same level as the nipples, has another. This area between the breasts is known as the middle cinnabar field. Roughly one inch above each nipple toward the corresponding shoulder there is another love point. One pair of love points is underneath each breast, under the breastbone; these love points should be pressed and stroked with the palm and felt lightly with the finger.

Groin ◈ Approximately two inches down the crease between the stomach and the thighs lie a pair of love points. Palpating them, by pushing lightly and stroking along the groin using the fingertips, can assuage frigidity and impotence.

Upper back ◈ The upper back contains four pairs of love points that may be stimulated for sexual energy. To find them, envisage on either side of the spine two parallel vertical lines. One is about one and one-half inches and the other about three inches from the spine. The top points align with the lower portion of the second thoracic vertebra (two vertebrae down from the large bone that protrudes at shoulder level when the head is bent forward, known as C-7). The bottom points line up with the lower part of the fifth thoracic vertebra (five vertebrae down from C-7). Press each point firmly for a few seconds, using the fingertips, and then stop. Go to the next point. Repeat the acupressure procedure a few times.

Lower back ❖ Directly under the second lumbar vertebra (located a bit below the back of the waist) on the spine is the *ming-men* (life gate). This is an important spot for sexual energy and the second center for a man's erection. Pressing on this love point firmly with the fingertips should bring about very satisfying results. Level with this point, there are two additional love points on either side of the spine. They are about one and one-half and three inches from the spine. They should be pressed together with the life gate.

Sacral-coccygeal area ❖ Along the sacrum, lined up in a V shape, there are eight love points that can be firmly pressed. There is a ninth spot on the tip of the coccyx.

Thighs and legs ❖ Midway between the kneecap and the groin on the front of each thigh lie two love points. Approximately two inches over the knee, where the muscles bulge slightly toward the inside, is another point. Press these firmly using the thumb.

Lower legs ❖ The most significant love point on the bottom portion of the leg is *san-yin-chiao* (intersection of three yins). It is on the inside of the shin, approximately three inches above the peak of the medial malleolus (anklebone) and beside the shinbone. Pressing here can cure impotence, frigidity, and early ejaculation.

EROTIC MASSAGE

Chinese erotic massage, over three thousand years old, is perhaps one of the most sexually exciting games in love play. It aims not so much at the muscles as at the Chi meridians as well as the central nervous system. These meridians control both body and mind. This august classical therapy, when used by a beloved mate for certain parts of the body, can increase the chemistry of desire wonderfully.

The intimate contact of hands and body is a form of indirect communication. It creates a rapport between the individuals. The partners in erotic massage are preferably naked or almost so. This allows the skin-to-skin exchange of life force and sexual energy. Any part of the body, barring the genitals, may be touched. All areas, except those that can be injured, such as the abdomen and breasts, may be massaged firmly. Gentle stroking of tender areas is used. The person getting the massage should lie on a floor mat, narrow table, daybed, or bed. A mattress is okay if it is extra firm.

Massage can be done with scented water or oil. If preferred, it is fine to use no lubricant at all. Furthermore, a home lubricant can be made with a mixture of two-thirds soybean oil, one-third sesame oil, and a fragrance such as lavender, chamomile, rose, sandalwood, or ylang-ylang. Sesame oil is helpful for the skin; ylang-ylang, which comes from a tropical Asian flower, is thought of as an aphrodisiac and assists blood pressure. Such oils can be purchased at Chinese grocery stores, natural-food shops, and pharmacies.

You should start the erotic massage with warming your hands, slapping them together, rubbing them vigorously while contracting

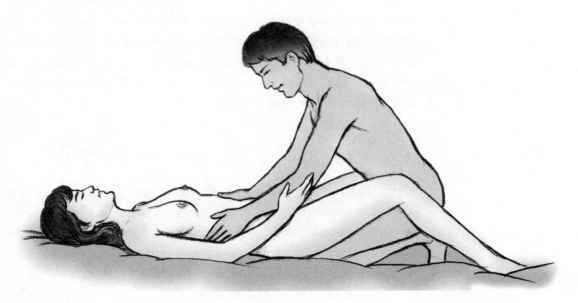

EROTIC MASSAGE

your perineum, and holding in a deep breath. Practice the art of moving your hand over the body without touching, slowly with intention focusing on the person and their skin and their whole body. Slowly come closer to the skin, lightly brushing just the hair at first and eventually barely touching the skin. Take your time, connect your hands to your heart. Pretend at first you are touching a newborn child and feel the quality of your touch shift. Open your heart and as you smile to your heart allow this "inner smile" to radiate out to your lover. Continue this "touching without touching" for ten or twenty minutes. When you do finally make contact with the skin, allow the hands to brush and drag lightly along, being soft without force. Eventually you can listen to your lover's body and slowly match his or her energy, applying more pressure in some areas and less in others. If you go inside yourself and listen, you will feel what your lover wants, and the erotic massage will unfold without instruction or memorizing moves or techniques. Use not only the pads of the fingers and palms but also the backs of the hands, the fingernails, and other parts of the body, avoiding the genitals for now. Ask for feedback, as everyone is different.

The massage can take about an hour. There is a shorter variety involving only the torso and thighs. This takes perhaps twenty minutes or less. The person being massaged should relax, eyes closed from time to time, and take slow, deep breaths using the diaphragm. There are numerous techniques for the actual massage. These include *effleurage* (long, rhythmic stroking), *tapotement* (patting, percussing), *pertrissage* (compressing, kneading), rubbing, pinching, pressing, scraping, grasping, hammering, shaking, and vibrating. The techniques use the thumb and finger pads, fingers, palms, palm edges, fists, soles, and elbows.

CARESSING THE MOON GROTTO

Caressing the Moon Grotto ◆ Being kissed and caressed by a lover is usually sufficient to arouse a woman so that her moon grotto becomes lubricated and her clitoris stiff. A woman's partner can easily check this by occasional short forays to the area of the vagina as he fondles her thighs and bottom. The clitoris is quite sensitive to touch. The shaft, instead of the sensitive tip, should be caressed. In

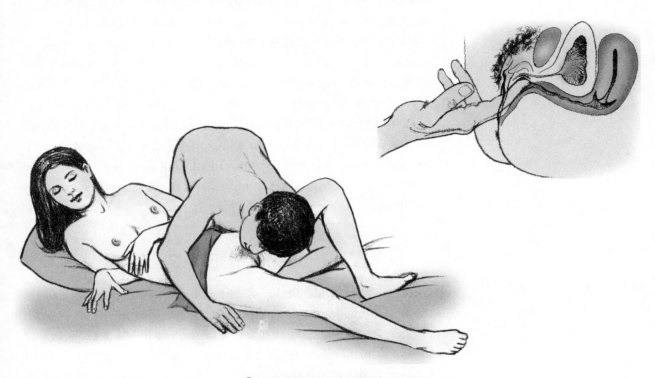

CARESSING THE MOON GROTTO

fact, some women can stand only the lightest touch to the tip, finding a heavy caress uncomfortable. By taking turns caressing the clitoris and then the vulva, first softly and then a little more firmly, a man may magnify the pleasure of his partner. If he strokes the labia minora, or inner lips, and then the edge of the vaginal opening with his middle and index fingers, more lubrication will flow. Taking these secretions with his fingers, he can rub the shaft of the clitoris with them. If the woman spreads her thighs wide, the classic texts tell us, she is responding positively to the love play. When her partner understands her signal, he can probe deeper into her moon grotto. Using one or two fingers to go deep enough to touch her flower heart (cervix) and lightly stroke it can increase her sensations.

If the woman's orgasm is the goal of the lovemaking, the man can bring this on by stimulating her clitoris. There are women capable of multiple orgasms by way of clitoral stimulation. Some particularly passionate women go from one orgasm to another for a relatively long time. Caressing her G-spot brings about a much more intense uterine orgasm. However, a lot of women appreciate a deep orgasm more during coitus. This is possible if the man knows the right positions and dynamics. The G-spot can be found by inserting the middle and index fingers about two inches inside the opening of the vagina. With finger pads facing the front wall of the vaginal canal, massage while exploring. A man can tell from the woman's reaction if he has found the spot (about the size of a bean). It may protrude a little when stimulated. Upon finding it, he can press the spot softly but rhythmically. Using the palm of the other hand to press down on her mons veneris at the same time, the man can increase the pressure on the spot.

CARESSING THE JADE STALK

Caressing the Jade Stalk ❖ Fondling a man's genitalia can be tricky. A lot depends on whether the man desires to ejaculate. If he doesn't, it is important that he be an expert in the techniques of orgasmic brinkmanship. If he is not, signals can be arranged so that the man can tell the woman when he is nearing ejaculation. A woman with experience can sense when the man is near the edge even without a signal. However, a man's ability to hold back may change from time to time, so it is always best to have some signals.

Caressing the jade stalk begins by gently stroking the perineum with the fingertips. Next the woman's fingers move softly to the back, bottom, and front of the scrotum with tickling but

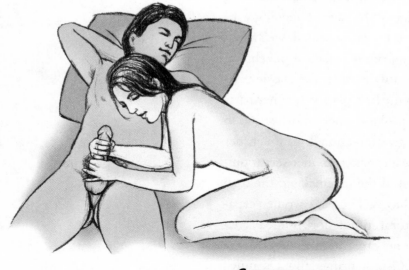

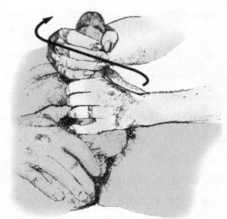

CARESSING THE JADE STALK

soothing caresses. Because the scrotum is the tenderest part of the male body, the woman should caress and tickle the testicles very gently. She should not pinch, squeeze, or nip at them. That is not love play and can cause serious pain, injury, or even disability. After the testicles have been caressed, the woman's fingers go to the man's erect penis. She grips it firmly near the tip with the palms and fingers and moves her grasp toward the base. This makes its skin more taut and reveals and tightens up the blood-filled glans, or head. She can stimulate the glans with the fingertips of her other hand with brisk, light rubbing. The undersurface of the erect penis is more sensitive than the top side, while the glans and the edge around its base are yet more sensitive. Most sensitive of all is the triangular, knot-shaped frenulum on the bottom side of the edge of the glans.

If the glans has leaked, the woman can apply the secretion with her fingertips in a circular motion around the glans. This can also be done with her own saliva. The caress can be varied by pumping the shaft up and down with her hand, but she must be careful the man does not ejaculate, unless this is intended. The stop-and-go method can assist the man in delaying or avoiding ejaculation, but it still gives him great pleasure and is tremendously arousing. If she is so moved, she can kiss the stalk while caressing it.

LOVE GAMES

Spring Butterfly ◈ In this love game the brush pen represents a springtime butterfly and the body a landscape of valleys and hills that is covered by flowers. The partner lies down with closed eyes and is completely relaxed. The end of the brush is placed here and there, mimicking a coquettish butterfly. First it is moved lightly over the hands and feet, and then it proceeds to arms, legs, and various parts of the body. The partner with the brush concentrates on sensitive areas like the fingertips, palms, insides of the elbows, armpits, soles, between the toes, behind the knees, and in particular, the insides of the thighs. Different portions of the face, including the lips, are teased next. The butterfly moves down the neck to the breasts, the abdomen, and the groin. The touches are delectable to the partner, especially because the partner does not know where the butterfly will land next. The light, galvanizing tickles created on the skin will

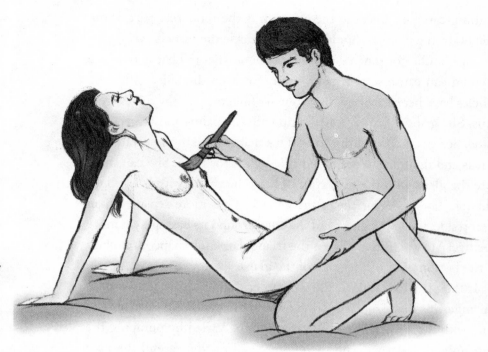

SPRING BUTTERFLY

probably bring forth a plea that the touches be firmer. The pleas should not be given in to until the damp landing is prepared. For this wonderful stage, the brush should first be dipped in a little aromatic oil. If the woman is the landscape, her areolae and nipples should be caressed with the oiled brush. First, go around and around and then flit between the breasts. After this, spread her legs and allow the butterfly to go along her perineum and vulva. Brush her clitoris next, first moving upward and next in a circular motion. For a man, brush his perineum and scrotum as well as the exposed glans. You may give your loved one a delightful and highly memorable hour with this marvelous game. A variation can be for a woman with long eyelashes to play the role of the spring butterfly by blinking. A man's moustache can be used for the same purpose. Such techniques may prove exhausting, however, if the entire landscape is covered.

Peacock Tease ✦ This game was invented hundreds of years ago when peacock feathers were used as a decoration of merit for service to the emperor. Lords interested in a different sort of merit used the peacock feather in a playful manner with their women. Today either partner can use the feather. Feathers from other birds such as ostriches, pheasants, storks, and even chickens can be used as well.

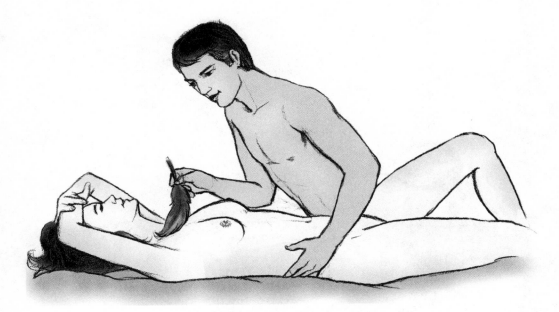

PEACOCK TEASE

You should remember, however, that feathers do not have as wide a variety of pressure as an artist's brush.

Spider's Legs ◆ There is a French love game called *pattes d'aragnee* where the fingertips and finger pads play on the partner's body hair, and sometimes the skin, with the lightest touches possible. As with the spring butterfly, the spider is capable of going all over the body.

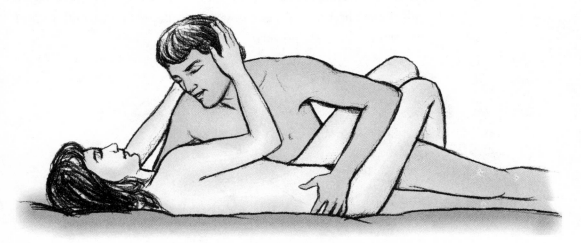

SPIDER'S LEGS

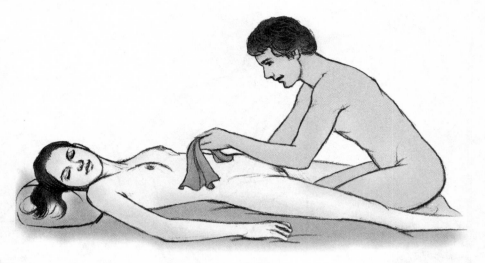

SILK TEASE

Silk Tease ◈ The best thing for this love game is a scarf or lingerie of real silk, but soft acetate will do. Nylon should not be used because it is too stiff. Ball up the scarf or other item a little in your hand, and use it to caress different parts of your partner's body. Silk provides a rich and luxurious sensation that is very different from that of brush pens or feathers.

Sniff-Kissing ◈ A sniff-kiss is best used if your partner's skin is perfumed slightly with crushed jasmine or tuberose, or if your partner's body gives forth its own sexual aroma. Start by inhaling and sniffing the breath of your lover. Nudge your nose on your partner's cheeks, eyelids, and neck, and proceed with the scented pilgrimage up the peaks and down the valleys. The natural odor of excited genitals is a powerful aphrodisiac.

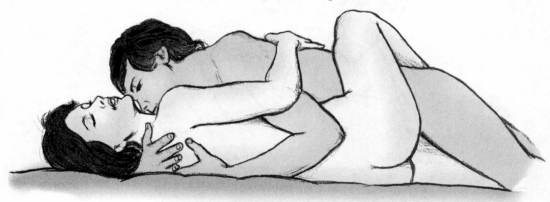

SNIFF-KISSING

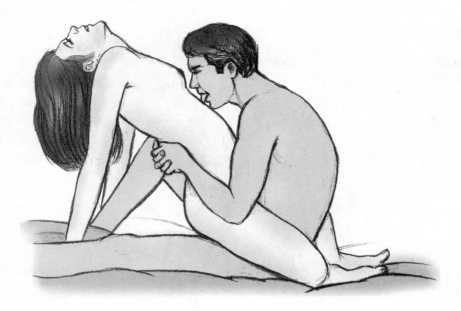

TONGUE SWEEP

Tongue Sweep ❖ This game usually starts quite naturally with a roving kiss. The tongue is showered on a partner with touches that can be everything from the lightest tickling with the end to a firm brushing with its rough surface. The ear cavity should be paid particular attention to, as well as under the chin and the palms and soles. Then go for the navel, breasts, and nipples, the inside of the thighs, and the perineum. A good tongue tease will use a lot of saliva and may result in drooling. Alternate the sweep with sniff-kisses.

THREE FOUNTAINS

Heavenly Fountain ❖ This is a love game that is done during deep kissing. It calls for stimulating the secretion of the lover's saliva and proceeding to drink it as a potion. While kissing, the tongue is used to caress the partner's tongue. After that, the tip of the tongue is swept over the roof of the partner's mouth beside the molars on both sides. The ducts leading from saliva glands are located here. In addition, sweep over the bottom of the partner's mouth along the inside of the teeth and particularly next to the tongue's root. Numerous ducts leading from saliva glands are located there. Such stimulation produces a great deal of saliva in

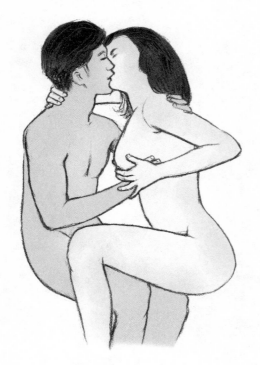

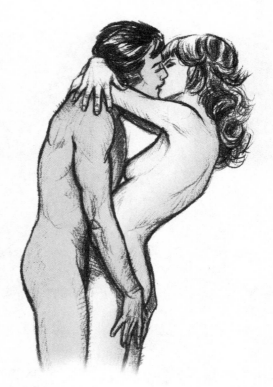

HEAVENLY FOUNTAIN

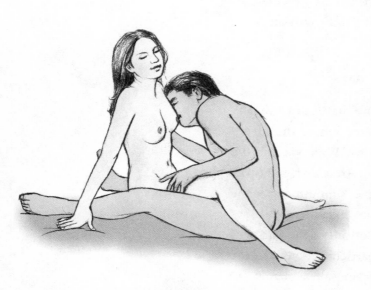

TWIN FOUNTAINS

the heavenly fountains of the partners. Ancient experts in the area of sex believed saliva was a sexual elixir. Nowadays, scientists believe it contains a sexual hormone whose taste is craved by the opposite sex. Drink it directly from the source.

Twin Fountains ❖ People everywhere kiss the female breasts. A male can give his love wonderful enjoyment by sucking on them as if he were a baby. Light and rhythmic sucking with occasional tickling with the tip of the tongue is one method. Gently squeeze as if milking them while sucking. The milk here is of a spiritual variety, unless, of course, the woman is nursing.

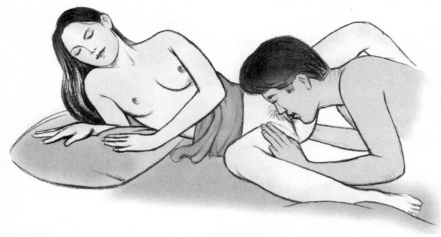

JADE FOUNTAIN

Jade Fountain   ❖   The Jade Fountain provides life nutrients for sexual alchemists to drink. Consequently, it is a serious undertaking. It is a most delightful event for love games. This is not an ordinary oral-genital kissing of the vulva. Rather, it involves the more complicated extraction of the jade essence (female ejaculate or ambrosia) from the fountain. For a man, this game has been likened to the splitting of a fresh pomegranate or the "peach of immortality," and the experience for the woman is beyond description.

The first thing necessary in the game is total cleanliness. Lying on her back, the woman bends her knees and spreads her thighs wide, with her buttocks near the edge of the bed. Another possibility is to slump in an armchair, with knees over the armrests. Facing her, the man kneels down. The partners could also lie in bed on their sides, or one on top, in opposite directions. These positions are excellent for this game or combined with Playing the Flute. Now the couple is ready to play the favorite French game of *soixante-neuf* (often called 69). The name itself shows us it is mutual oral-genital play.

First the man kisses the partner's mons veneris. Following that he opens the outside lips of her genitalia with his fingers, and kisses the inner lips. The tongue should be used to stroke the inner lips, and by this stage they should already be engorged with blood. Thinking of the vulva as the sides of a boat, the urethra, the vaginal orifice, and the four vestibular glands are on the bottom. Take the tip of the tongue and sweep up and down the bottom of the boat.

Drive the tongue into the vagina and then remove it. Repeat this rhythmically. Gradually, the man should go on to the clitoral area. Kiss the tiny button with your lips. Suck it ever so gently and tickle the tip with your tongue like a teasing butterfly. The rough surface of the tongue licks up from the bottom of the clitoral shaft. Alternate between caressing the clitoris and the vulva. Concentrate on things that elicit your partner's most excited responses. This will inescapably cause the jade fountain to bubble over with the jade essence of the vestibular glands and the grotto well. Occasionally it produces some interesting sounds too.

Playing the Flute ◈ This game, too, as with the Jade Fountain, necessitates meticulous personal cleanliness and a great degree of delicacy. There are women who love it, but others do not care for it. This is often because of the hazards involved. First there is the gag reflex if the man goes deep into the throat. There is also the possibility of accidental swallowing of the semen if the man cannot or will not practice orgasmic brinkmanship. With practice and cooperation, though, everything is easily under control. Other issues are strictly a matter of personal taste.

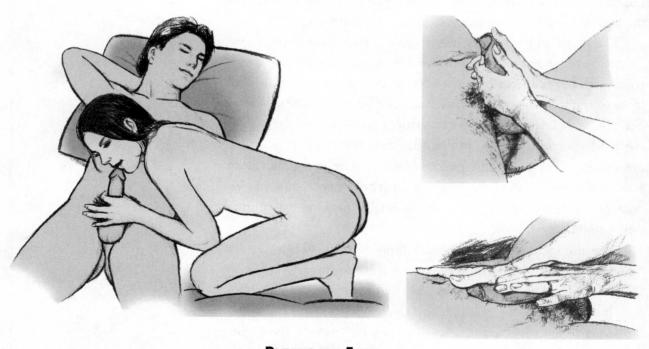

PLAYING THE FLUTE

It is best to begin the game with the woman kissing the man's perineum and scrotum. Following that is the flute playing. The woman should hold the base of the jade flute firmly with one hand so that it stands up. A series of light kisses should be given to the glans. Then the woman holds the glans in her mouth by surrounding the ridge with her lips. She licks the glans, especially the small urethral opening, with the tip of her tongue. Next she should purse her mouth into a tight O shape and picture it as the opening to her grotto. She moves her mouth up and down and lets her partner move the flute in and out. At the same time, her fingers play with his perineum and scrotum. It should be kept in mind that the most sensitive part is the top third of the flute, which includes the head.

A lot of men, perhaps for psychological reasons more than for physical pleasure, like their partners to "deep-throat" the flute. When the tip of the flute contacts the woman's throat, it normally activates the gag reflex. However, by practicing a gradual deepening method, a woman can accept the entire flute easily. Playing the flute, especially deep-throat music, can cause a man to ejaculate in the woman's mouth. There are women who avidly swallow the potion. Scientists claim it is clean and harmless. The ancient belief was that it is beneficial. Some women, however, do not like this. It is possible, of course, for a woman to keep the fluid in her mouth and spit it out. Another possibility is to arrange ahead of time for the man to signal when he is on the edge.

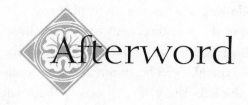

Afterword

This book on sexual reflexology is really a book about energy, the most basic and powerful form of human energy: sexual energy. Without sexual energy none of us would be here. There would be no book to write and no one to read it. Sexual energy, the primal union of yin and yang forces, drives the universe, and yet most people approach it without much understanding. It brings ecstasy and deep joy but also causes deep pain and heartache from lack of proper knowledge. It can heal our bodies, or it can cause sickness, confusion, and disease.

Through study of sexual reflexology it is possible to understand sexual energy from an entirely new perspective and level . . . but where do you go from here? What do you do now? Nothing! That's the Way. That's the Tao. It may seem confusing to you now, but after you try some of the concepts and practices in this book, it will begin to make sense to you. You will discover Nondoing or Doing Nothing (the Taoists call it Wu Wei), which may be translated as "effortless action" or "correct action" or just "going with the flow." Correct action (Wu Wei) is the letting go of your will, which is action on your part. As you let go, the sexual energy (Chi) flows through you, and eventually, by practicing the formulas (correct action), you will connect with that energy and become one with it. And that's the Tao. The information in this book may be studied and comprehended by our mind, but it is only when these concepts come to live in our bodies that we really begin to understand it.

The Tao says there are three ways of enlightenment. The first way is one of prayer and worship; you can achieve it, but you don't know when, why, or how. The second way is one of good works and service, but again, you don't know when, why, or how. The third way is the Way of the Tao, which is one of knowledge and wisdom. You know when, why, and how, because it is an alchemical process on a molecular level working with the highest form of energy (sexual energy) in the body, and this will become clear to you as you practice. You will know when to be hard and when to be soft. That's wisdom, and that's the Tao.

We thank you for your time and attention. We trust you will see your sexual experience a little clearer now and begin to understand the way of your sexuality and begin to incorporate these new ways of understanding human sexual energy into your life, a process that takes many years. It is the work of a lifetime. So play with these new concepts, new positions, new attitudes, and new understandings, but be easy on yourself. There is no right or wrong way to get in touch with your own personal sexual energy. It takes time, patience, humor, and love. We hope you will take these qualities, bring them to your sexual practice, and enjoy a whole new way of relating to yourself and your sexual partners that will bring you many years of peace and joy.

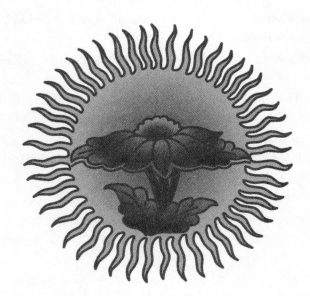

PATIENCE, HUMOR, AND LOVE

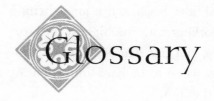

Glossary

Arcane Maid / Elemental Maid / Plain Girl All refer to a legendary young woman whose knowledge of sexual matters was transcribed to a handbook intended to enhance the health and longevity of ancient emperors.

Channel A path that the Chi/energy takes as it moves in the body.

Chi muscle See PC muscle.

Cranial pump Located at the base of the skull, at the occipital ridge.

Dual cultivation Practice with a partner—exchanging energy.

G-spot Located usually in (though not limited to) the upper vagina, one to one and one-half inches in. More easily distinguished in an aroused state as the periurethral sponge swells and the G-spot is then felt as a ridgelike spot or like a flower bud starting to open.

Hui-yin Acupuncture point located at the perineum.

Lower Tan Tien Tan Tien means elixir field. The Lower Tan Tien is found at the navel center area.

Meridians Clear and defined energy paths in the body that Chi/energy flows through.

Ming-men The "door of life" (not to be mistaken for the "gate of life & death"), located slightly below and between the kidneys.

PC Chi muscle A muscle in a figure-8 shape that is connected both to the pubic bone and coccyx bone. The mid-point is at the perineum, between the genitals and anus.

PC (pubococcygeus) muscle See PC Chi muscle.

Pelvic diaphragm Also known as the levator ani muscle. Very important to the health and vitality of all internal organs as it works like the 'floor' of the pelvis/torso.

Perineum External region between the genitals and anus, location of the energy point "gate of life and death." Vital to sexual practice.

Reverse breathing Pulling the abdomen inwards upon the inhale, and relaxing outwards on the exhale.

Sacral pump Small movements of the sacrum that pump the spinal fluid up the spine.

Single cultivation Practice done alone, with no partner and no energy exchange.

Universal Tao Mantak Chia's complete system of Taoist Practices.

Urogenital diaphragm Small diaphragm attached to the bladder and internal genitals. Responsible for keeping the bladder and internal sex organs in place. Not to be mistaken for the pelvic diaphragm, which is much bigger.

TAOIST TERMS

These are ancient terms and can have more than one meaning.

Baby palace, ovarian palace Uterus

Cinnabar field Three fingers below the navel, not a fixed point, but an area that includes up, down, left and right

Cinnabar grotto Uterus

Flower heart G-spot

Gate Vagina

Grain seed Vagina

Grotto Vagina

Infant girl Vestibular glands between the labia minora

Jade essence Female ejaculate

Jade flute / jade stalk / jade stem Penis

Jade gate Vagina

Jewel terrace Clitoris

Lute strings Frenulum of clitoris; one inch inside the vagina

Mixed rock Four inches deep in the vagina

Moon grotto Vagina

Scarlet chamber Vagina

Scarlet pearls Labia minora

Scented mouse Vulva

Wheat buds Labia minora; two inches deep

Yang peak Penis

Yang terrace Mouth of uterus/cervix

Yin Vagina

Yin gate Labia minora

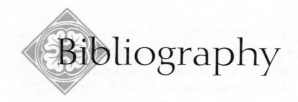# Bibliography

Beinfield, Harriet, and Efrem Korngold. *Between Heaven and Earth.* New York: Ballantine Books, 1992.

Chang, Dr. Stephen T. *The Great Tao.* San Francisco: Tao Publishing, 1985.

Chia, Mantak. *Healing Love through the Tao: Cultivating Female Sexual Energy.* Chiang Mai, Thailand: Universal Tao Publications, 2002.

Chia, Mantak. *Chi Nei Tsang II: Internal Organ Chi Massage Chasing the Winds.* Chiang Mai, Thailand: Universal Tao Publications, 2000.

Chia, Mantak. *Taoist Secrets of Love: Cultivating Female Sexual Energy.* Huntington, N.Y.: Healing Tao Books, 1986.

Chia, Mantak. *Taoist Ways to Transform Stress into Vitality.* Huntington, N.Y.: Healing Tao Books, 1985.

Chia, Mantak, and Douglas Abram. *The Multi-Orgasmic Couple.* San Francisco: Harper Collins, 2000.

Chia, Mantak, and Douglas Abram. *The Multi-Orgasmic Man.* San Francisco: HarperCollins, 1996.

Chia, Mantak, and Juan Li. *Inner Structure of Tai Chi.* Huntington, N.Y.: Healing Tao Books, 1996.

Chia, Mantak with Michael Winn. *Taoist Secrets of Love: Cultivating Male Sexual Energy.* New York: Aurora Press, 1984.

Chu, Valentin. *Yin-Yang Butterfly: Ancient Chinese Sexual Secrets for Western Lovers.* New York: G. P. Putnam's Sons, 1985.

Garbourg, Paula. *Self Healing: The Secrets of the Ring Muscles.* Fort Lauderdale, Fla.: Peleg Publishers, 1991.

Sachs, Bob. *The Complete Guide to Nine Star Ki.* Rockport, Mass.: Element, 1996.

Tortora, Gerard J. and Sandra Reynolds Grabowski. *Introduction to the Human Body: The Essentials of Anatomy and Physiology*, Fifth Edition. Hoboken, N.J.: John Wiley and Sons, 2000.

White, Suzanne. *The New Astrology.* New York: St. Martin's Press, 1992.

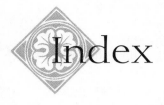

Index

Page numbers in italics refer to illustrations. Page numbers in bold refer to glossary definitions.

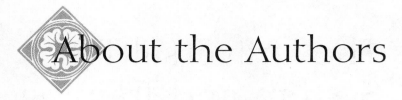

About the Authors

MANTAK CHIA

Mantak Chia has been studying the Taoist approach to life since childhood. His mastery of this ancient knowledge, enhanced by his study of other disciplines, has resulted in the development of the Universal Tao System, which is now being taught throughout the world.

Mantak Chia was born in Thailand to Chinese parents in 1944. When he was six years old, he learned from Buddhist monks how to sit and "still the mind." While in grammar school he learned traditional Thai boxing, and soon went on to acquire considerable skill in Aikido, Yoga, and Tai Chi. His studies of the Taoist way of life began in earnest when he was a student in Hong Kong, ultimately leading to his mastery of a wide variety of esoteric disciplines. To better understand the mechanisms behind healing energy, he also studied Western anatomy and medical sciences.

Master Chia has taught his system of healing and energizing practices to tens of thousands of students and trained more than two thousand instructors and practitioners throughout the world. He has established centers for Taoist study and training in many countries around the globe. In June 1990 he was honored by the International Congress of Chinese Medicine and Qi Gong (Chi Kung), which named him the Qi Gong Master of the Year.

WILLIAM U. WEI

William Wei grew up in the Midwest region of the United States. He began studying under Master Mantak Chia in the early 1980s and later became a Senior Instructor of the Universal Tao, specializing in one-on-one training. He has taught with Master Chia in over thirty countries and manages a variety of Universal Tao projects. William Wei has written five books of Taoist poetry as well as the instructive book *Living in the Tao*.

The Universal Tao System and Training Center

THE UNIVERSAL TAO SYSTEM

The ultimate goal of Taoist practice is to transcend physical boundaries through the development of the soul and the spirit within the human. That is also the guiding principle behind the Universal Tao, a practical system of self-development that enables individuals to complete the harmonious evolution of their physical, mental, and spiritual bodies. Through a series of ancient Chinese meditative and internal energy exercises, the practitioner learns to increase physical energy, release tension, improve health, practice self-defense, and gain the ability to heal oneself and others. In the process of creating a solid foundation of health and well-being in the physical body, the practitioner also creates the basis for developing his or her spiritual potential by learning to tap into the natural energies of the Sun, Moon, Earth, Stars and other environmental forces.

The Universal Tao practices are derived from ancient techniques rooted in the processes of nature. They have been gathered and integrated into a coherent, accessible system for well-being that works directly with the life force, "Chi," flowing through the meridian system of the body.

Master Chia has spent years developing and perfecting techniques for passing these traditional practices to students around the world through ongoing classes, workshops, private instruction and healing sessions, as well as books and video and audio products. Further information can be obtained at www.universal-tao.com.

UNIVERSAL TAO CENTER

The Tao Garden Resort and Training Center in northern Thailand is the home of Master Chia and serves as the worldwide headquarters for Universal Tao activities. This integrated wellness, holistic health, and training center is situated on eighty acres surrounded by the beautiful Himalayan foothills near the historic walled city of Chiang Mai. The serene setting includes flower and herb gardens ideal for meditation, open-air Simple Chi Kung pavilions, and a health and fitness spa offering treatments.

The Center also offers classes year-round, as well as summer and winter retreats. It can accommodate 200 students, and group leasing can be arranged. For more information you may fax the Center at (66)(53) 495-852, or email:

universaltao@universal-tao.com.

BOOKS OF RELATED INTEREST

THE SEXUAL TEACHINGS OF THE WHITE TIGRESS
Secrets of the Female Taoist Masters
by Hsi Lai

THE SEXUAL TEACHINGS OF THE JADE DRAGON
Taoist Methods for Male Sexual Revitalization
by Hsi Lai

QIGONG TEACHINGS OF A TAOIST IMMORTAL
The Eight Essential Exercises of Master Li Ching-yun
by Stuart Alve Olson

CHI KUNG
The Chinese Art of Mastering Energy
by Yves Réquéna

THE REFLEXOLOGY MANUAL
An Easy-to-Use Illustrated Guide to the Healing
Zones of the Hands and Feet
by Pauline Wills

SHARP SPEAR, CRYSTAL MIRROR
Martial Arts in Women's Lives
by Stephanie T. Hoppe

TANTRIC SECRETS FOR MEN
What Every Woman Will Want Her Man to Know
about Enhancing Sexual Ecstasy
by Kerry Riley with Diane Riley, co-creators of
The Secrets of Sacred Sex *video*

**SEXUAL SECRETS: TWENTIETH
ANNIVERSARY EDITION**
The Alchemy of Ecstasy
by Nik Douglas and Penny Slinger

Inner Traditions • Bear & Company
P.O. Box 388
Rochester, VT 05767
1-800-246-8648